Dep:

Blues

How to conquer sadness, loneliness, and despair –
you <u>can</u> live a happy life!

by
John H. Clark III

www.depressionblues.net
www.johnclarkbooks.com
www.johnhenryiii.com

Dedication

This book is dedicated to my father, John Henry Clark Jr., a good man who always worked hard to support his family, but also suffered from severe depression and lacked the emotional resources to give and receive love and affection.

published by: johnclarkbooks

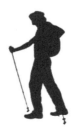

Table of contents

Introduction

I will never forget the day I called the local offices of a state mental health agency.

A young lady answered, and I told her I needed help.

"What's wrong?" she asked me.

"I feel like killing myself," I said.

"Well," she responded, then after a long pause. "Um, that's not good."

That's not good?

No shit, lady, I thought, and hung up the phone.

That's not good. Hell, I knew that before I called.

By this time in my life – 32 years old, newly divorced, flat broke, living alone on the floor of a cheap apartment with no furniture, self-medicating my way through the day – I was at my wit's end, hanging onto my evaporating sanity by a steadily unraveling thread.

I do not think I really wanted to kill myself, but I was completely and utterly miserable, hopeless, with no end to it in sight. Every day was an absolute drudgery. What I really wanted was to collapse somewhere in public, just pass out right there on the sidewalk, and have someone pick me up – literally or figuratively – and take me to a hospital, where I presumably would be taken care of, comforted, and loved.

That never happened, but fortunately, something else did; a true miracle that pulled me back from the edge, and started me on the road to recovery and building a new life. I will recount the details of that unforgettable experience later in this book.

Suffice it to say, I know firsthand about depression.

My father has suffered from depression the better part of his life, and apparently this is one of the things he handed down to the next generation. All three of his kids have various emotional issues, but I am not sure whether those issues are the result of nature or nurture. Did we actually inherit his depressive and pessimistic mind as a result of genetics? Were we born with a predisposition for mental illness already lurking in our DNA? Or was it a behavior, an attitude, a self-destructive way of thinking that we learned as a result of being around him throughout our formative years?

One thing I will always remember about my old man is following behind him, walking into church on Sunday mornings. From the dark asphalt parking lot, up the gray concrete sidewalk steps, through the door, there was a long carpeted hallway lined on both sides with meeting rooms, classrooms and offices leading to the side door of the chapel and the rest of the building, and I can still see a picture in my mind of other men greeting him with a smile and a vigorous handshake.

"How you doin' today, brother Clark?"

"Terrible, how about yourself?"

That was his standard answer. Now, he may have been kidding, but I honestly don't think so.

Throughout my life – even long after the miracle happened – I have been on an emotional rollercoaster, of sorts. Up and down; around and around. I have read books, listened to tapes and CDs, gone to counseling, undergone hypnosis, acupuncture, reiki, taken yoga classes, meditated, done Chinese qigong, taken four or five different types of medications, tried to drown my sorrows in wine and women.

None of those things ever helped.

So considering my struggles, who am I to write a book and tell you how to feel better? What makes me qualified for such a thing? Well, because I have been down nearly every road already, tried all kinds of avenues to magically flip a switch and turn myself into a happy person.

That makes me an expert – not a mental health expert, but an expert of my own story.

In this book, I'm going to share my travels in and out of insanity. Some of it is going to be ugly, but I also am going to share how I came out the other side, and am now living a fairly happy and productive life, filled with love and friends, a comfortable lifestyle, and hope for the future.

Depression is a terrible thing, but it can be overcome.

I promise you that. It can be overcome.

Chapter One

A lot of my childhood, I do not remember anymore.

We lived in a small, three-bedroom, frame house on a corner lot in a tidy, new subdivision on the northwest side of Houston, Texas, not far from the railroad tracks and a branch of Buffalo Bayou. I can remember being in my bed at night, listening to the train whistles blow through the still night air.

I was the oldest child, followed by my sister and then my brother. We were fairly happy kids, as I recall, playing outside after school and all day long on the weekends with the other neighborhood kids: hide-n-go-seek, tag, chase, football in the street, baseball in someone's front yard or down at the park a block away, riding bicycles, skateboards, roller skating up and down the sidewalk, flagging down the jingle-jangling ice cream truck.

Your basic all-American stuff.

When it started getting dark, it was time to go home. Sometimes, we'd hear a loud, long whistle from dad's pursed lips, and that meant it was time to get home – now.

Discipline was harsh in our house; hugs and kisses were non-existent.

There was no such thing as time-out, or grounding, or taking away privileges in those days. Hell, there was no negotiation, no argument, no talking back. Are you kidding?

When you broke a rule or did something stupid, punishment was swift, and came at the end of a leather belt. Lay across the side of mom and dad's bed, and take a series of wallops on the backside. Try and block or dodge those stinging blows, and they might land on another part of the anatomy. Often did.

My little brother usually got the worst of it. I remember listening to him crying, "That's enough! That's enough!" while I counted the number of times he got hit, over and over and over. The counting continued well into the twenties, always. This happened a lot. Daily sometimes.

If that sort of thing were happening today, my mother especially would have been arrested for child abuse.

But that was the world we lived in, and whippings were not unusual. It was a common sight, for instance, to see the kid right next door, Dennis, come busting out the front screen door of his house, hands covering his rear end, crying "No, no, no," with his mom in hot pursuit, brandishing a switch pulled from a tree in the yard and chasing him down the sidewalk for a little corporal punishment.

I also remember Dennis taking dumps in the flower beds in front of his house. Turds in the dirt. Not sure if those switchings had anything to do with the poor kid crapping outside all the time, but it kind of seems like there might be a connection.

At school, there was paddling, as well. In third grade, the teacher was a big woman who laid you across her lap and spanked you with her hand, in front of the whole class. In junior high and high school, coaches lined up the athletes on report card day and gave swats with a wooden board for bad grades. A trip to the principal's office often resulted in at least one painful pop on the butt.

When I was a senior, I was tardy to my first period class every day. After the tardies reached the magic number – I don't remember now what that number was – my teacher, Mr. Watts, offered me the choice of going to the office, or taking a swat from him.

It was pretty much six of one or a half-dozen of the other, so I chose the swat. I'd come to class late, Mr. Watts – a very nice man and respected teacher for whom I hold not one iota of ill will – would grab his board from a desk drawer, and we'd go out into the hallway, over to the stairwell, conveniently a short distance away. This is how it was done in those days.

We would walk down to the staircase, where I'd bend over and touch the first or second step with my fingertips, and … boom! The paddle connected, the sound echoed off the walls, and then it was back to class, me pretending it was not that bad; my butt cheeks burning for a few minutes.

Like I said, that was normal stuff, and nothing that scarred me for life. That's the way it was back in the day.

What did scar me for life was the lack of love and affection inside my house.

From the outside, I'm sure ours seemed like the all-American little family, but inside was a different story. I rarely saw either one of my parents show any affection toward the other. They never sat on the sofa together, talking, laughing, holding hands. I never walked in on them hugging and kissing in the kitchen, or anywhere else. Never heard one say "I love you" to the other. The only time I ever saw them even touch each other was when the old man left for work in the morning. Mama would follow him to the front door, where he turned around and gave her the perfunctory peck on the lips.

Unfortunately, that lack of overt affection also extended to the children.

We were not a huggy-kissy family, to say the least.

For some reason, even though I don't really remember my mother ever telling me she loved me when I was a kid, somehow I knew she did. Maybe simply because she was my mother, she took care of me, and I felt safe around her. I don't know. She had her own issues – one of which I found out later was being trapped in an unhappy marriage – but she liked to have fun, and she was a good mom. She did not work outside the home for a long time, but when she could scrape enough money together, she'd take us to the movies, bowling, across town to visit her sister, and to spend weekends and holidays at my grandparents' house in the piney east Texas woods surrounding Sam Rayburn lake.

My mother liked to bake, and I remember every year making Christmas cookies, rolling out sheets of homemade dough on flour-dusted wax paper, cutting out various shapes like candy canes, stars, reindeer, Santa Clauses. Using an old-fashioned pastry bag to squeeze out sweet, sugary icing after the cookies were baked and cooled, then adding sprinkles, red hot candies, and other decorations.

At my mother's funeral, I mentioned how she taught me to make a cherry pie, my all-time favorite, completely from scratch. Same thing with cakes, although my job with cakes was usually to lick the mixing bowl and, hopefully, at least one beater after the cake batter was poured into the pan.

Wonderful memories.

I never doubted my mother's love.

My father, on the other hand, was a completely different story.

Dad was a provider. He was head of the family, earned the money, controlled the purse strings, and ruled with an iron fist. His word was law, and there was no disputing it. In his world, kids were meant to be seen and not heard – literally. That's the way it was. To argue with him, or even attempt to talk back, was unheard of in our family. He was, to say the least, not very approachable.

I do remember him telling me he loved me, but that was when I was twenty-six years old, married with a child of my own, and by then, I really didn't want to hear it.

Let me explain.

We were standing in my second-floor apartment, rays of the setting sun streaming through the living room window – my parents were divorced by then – and my dad was handing me a check to help with my first semester's tuition at the University of Houston, which back then was a couple of hundred bucks or something. I had decided to go back to school, and he said he wanted to help out.

Back when I was a senior in high school, he told me one time that he would pay for my college, but I had to continue to live at home while I went. That was not an attractive offer. But now, he wanted to keep his part of the bargain.

As my old man started to leave, he suddenly stepped forward, put his arms around me and said, "I love you."

My reaction?

Tears and a warm father-and-son embrace as I finally heard, at long last, the words I'd waited for all my life?

Hardly.

I froze, with my arms down at my sides and just stood there.

Uncomfortable.

Really, it kind of pissed me off. All I could think was, "Where in the hell was this when I was ten or eleven years old?"

Sure, my old man did a lot of things for me when I was a kid, like taking me to the hardware store for lumber to build a cool set of wooden stilts that were so tall you had to prop them up against the side of the house and climb up to start walking, installing a regulation-height basketball goal out alongside the driveway, building a red-dirt pitching mound and home plate in the backyard, signing me up for Little League, and even coaching some of my teams.

I didn't understand at the time that was his way of telling me – showing me – that he loved me. A hug, or even a pat on the back once in a while, sure would have been nice.

A kid needs to hear the words.

I remember my first year in peewee football, my very first practice. I was eight years old, and I'm sure there was calisthenics, running, tackling practice and such, but the thing I will never forget about my first-ever football practice is the scrimmage at the end.

I have no idea how they sorted things out, but I think basically it was 'A Team' offense, which included the players from the year before who knew what they were doing, against everybody else.

That's how it was back in the day. They wanted to see who had a natural instinct for the game, and who did not. Which ones didn't mind sticking their head in there and making some contact.

For whatever reason, they lined me up at left defensive end, and it might have been the first play, but I'll never forget – a kid named Steve, one of the veterans and an incredible athlete, took a handoff from the quarterback and headed straight up the middle. This kid was fast and tough, both arms wrapped around the football, knees driving hard, and he appeared to have clear sailing through everybody, until I ran across and launched myself horizontally into his right side, wrapped my arms around his waist and flattened him.

I didn't think much about it – that was what they told me to do, after all – but when I went back to my position and knelt down to get ready for the next play, a couple of the coaches came over with big smiles on their faces and slapped me on the helmet a couple of times, told me way to go, way to hit, stuff like that.

My old man was there, but never said anything. Not even later, on the way home.

When I was eleven, I wanted more than anything in the world to make the Little League all-star baseball team. My dad was a coach in our league, and so he went to the meeting where all the coaches picked the players who would be on the team.

I was already in bed when he got home from the meeting, and I heard him call me into the dining room. He was sitting in a chair, my mother was standing nearby in the kitchen, and I walked over and stood in front of him, and he said, "You didn't make it."

That was it. You didn't make it. Nothing like, "You did a great job this year, son, and I think you should have made it. I'm really proud of you." Maybe a hug, as well. A handshake. Something.

Nope. Not my old man. I stood there in my Fruit of the Looms, tears rolling down my face, and he told me to go back to bed.

A year later, I did in fact make the all-star team, but that dream come true proved to be the beginning of the end to our relationship for a long time. I'll tell that story later.

It wasn't until I was somewhere in my forties that my dad told me he was proud of me, and even then, he apparently couldn't spit out the actual words, so he typed them up in a letter. As was the case with the hug and the "I love you" years before, I was not overly impressed.

So, I grew up in an emotionally stilted environment. Our family never talked about much of anything, but especially not about feelings.

My sister told me once after we were grown that she went to our dad one time about a problem she was having – those two were always very close – and his advice to her was this: "Well, don't feel that way."

Simple. Problem solved. Feeling bad? Hurt, anxious, afraid, angry, sad? The solution is simple.

Just don't feel that way.

Thanks, pops.

To this day, I have a hard time understanding my emotions. Basically, I know that I either feel bad or I feel good. That's about it. Ask me to explain why I feel a certain way, try to get to the root of the problem, and I have a really hard time. Usually, I can't do it. I don't have a clue.

Chapter Two

According to the famed Mayo Clinic, depression is defined as "a mood disorder that causes a persistent feeling of sadness and loss of interest. Also called major depressive disorder or clinical depression, it affects how you feel, think, and behave and can lead to a variety of emotional and physical problems. You may have trouble doing normal day-to-day activities, and sometimes you may feel as if life isn't worth living."

A lot of people going through the normal ups and downs of life experience bouts of sadness or "the blues" from time to time. It is when those occasional feelings of despair and emptiness take hold and begin to affect your life that it is time to take a look at the possibility of having a more serious problem.

Symptoms of depression include such things as:

- Excessive fatigue; lack of energy.
- Trouble sleeping, or sleeping too much.
- Feelings of hopelessness, helplessness, sadness, loneliness. The idea that things are never going to get any better, so what is the point of going on?
- Losing interest in activities that once were sources of great pleasure, including sports, hobbies, and sex.
- Self-medicating, with alcohol or drugs, for example.
- Overeating, or lack of appetite.
- Excessive feelings of guilt and regret; focusing on past failures or mistakes; blaming yourself for things that are not your fault.
- Difficulty concentrating, remembering things, and making decisions.
- Unexplained physical problems, such as headaches, backaches.
- Frequent thoughts of suicide.

I am quite familiar with some of those: hopelessness, irritability, loss of interest in pleasurable activities, sleeping too much, not getting enough sleep, lack of energy, feelings of worthlessness, fixating on past failures, tired of living.

Where does that all come from? When did it all start?

In spite of my upbringing – which was not horrible, by any means, especially compared to what some kids go through – I would not describe myself as a depressed kid. A better description would probably be … intense.

All our old home movies are long gone, destroyed by wind and rain and critters in a dilapidated house that my old man bought about the time I graduated from high school. It was a fixer-upper that never got fixed up after he had it moved out to a four-acre lot in the country. He still owns the place, but nobody has lived there for years, and time and neglect have nearly destroyed it completely.

But I remember one old movie that shows me on a swing set in our backyard – probably about age five – and I'm pumping that swing back and forth so furiously it's a wonder that the whole thing did not either become airborne, or come tumbling down.

When all the other kids in the neighborhood got new roller skates and were happily cruising up and down the sidewalk, I was practicing inside our closed-door, one-car garage, going round and round, bouncing off the walls and a large chest freezer for I don't know how long, until I thought I was good enough to go outside and skate with everybody else.

As far back as I can remember, I have always been a raging perfectionist. I'm not as bad as I used to be – I can even put a postage stamp on an envelope now without having to line it up perfectly square in the corner – but I still have tendencies.

When I was eight years old, I started playing sports. First came football, then Little League baseball. I was not a natural at either one, but I was athletic and coordinated, and I worked hard and I caught on quickly. I absolutely loved sports, but I had a big problem with losing.

It wasn't until I was a grown man that I read about a saying from the great Austin golf instructor Harvey Penick that went something like this: "You are who you are; you ain't what you do!"

I have always judged my self-worth by my accomplishments. As a kid, it was sporting accomplishments. As an adult, professional accomplishments. I never understood that who I am and what I do are two separate things. I understand that a little better now, but I still have a hard time sometimes separating the two.

When I was fifteen years old, I quit playing sports altogether. I was kind of burnt-out at that point, had suffered some pretty serious injuries, and we had some real assholes for coaches at my high school. I was getting to the age where I didn't want people telling me what to do, and I think one of the main reasons I quit everything was because I knew it would devastate my old man. I really hated him then, and I knew this would be a punishing blow.

What happened between my dad and me? Why did I now despise the man who was once my hero? I'll tell you why.

Like I said, I spent all my life trying to make the guy proud. If he'd just one time said something positive or encouraging, who knows what might have happened? I'd run through walls for someone who gave me a pat on the back.

Remember when I talked about the Little League all-stars? Well, after my eleven-year-old season, I went on a tear of practicing in my backyard. Dad had built a regulation pitching mound back there, along with a makeshift backstop and a home plate, exactly forty-six feet away from the mound. It stretched pretty much from one fence line to the other.

I was out there every day, throwing baseballs, retrieving them, hustling back to the mound and throwing some more.

My twelve-year-old season, I was the top pitcher in our league, threw two no-hitters and never lost a game. I not only made all-stars, I was the number one pitcher on the all-star team, which included some excellent little athletes, many of whom went on to star in high school and even college sports.

I was on top of the world.

Then came the night of our first game in the local tournament that would eventually lead to the annual Little League World Series in Williamsport, Pennsylvania. Big stuff for a kid.

I was the starting pitcher, and it was standing-room-only, with a huge crowd on hand. We were home team, and so took the field first. I basically had two pitches, a decent but not overpowering fastball and a wicked curveball that I could throw inside, outside, high, low, anywhere I wanted it to go. My curve was nearly unhittable.

The first pitch of the game was a fastball, low and down the middle. The kid swatted it on the ground right at our shortstop, who failed to get his glove all the way down, and the ball went right through him, between his feet, out into left field. Runner on first.

Second pitch, identical to the first, with the same result. Another fastball, low and down the middle. Batter slaps it right at the shortstop, who does not get his glove down all the way; ball rolls out to left field. Runners on first and second, no outs.

Oh, shit.

Their dugout and their fans were going wild, screaming and cheering, smelling blood in the water.

I'd seen enough.

Our catcher gave me the sign for another fastball, and I shook him off. He put down two fingers, signal for a curveball, and I nodded my head, wound up and delivered. Strike one. Catcher signals again for a fastball. Nope, I shook my head, until he flashed two fingers.

Another curveball. Strike two. Another curveball. Strike three.

OK, that's better.

From then on, every pitch I threw for the rest of the game was a curveball. Nobody else got on base, and we were winning the game 4-0 going into the fifth inning. By then, two things were happening. First, their best hitters were coming up to bat for the second and third time, and they were figuring out what I was doing. Second, twisting off curveballs puts a strain on your arm, and I had thrown a lot of them.

They stopped swinging at bad pitches, and I stopped being able to hit my spots. I started walking people.

I walked three in a row, filling the bases, and I kept throwing curveballs. I was afraid to throw another fastball, after those two errors to start the game. After I walked five guys in a row, our coach took me out and put in a fresh pitcher, who promptly shut them down and preserved our 4-2 lead.

I watched the rest of the game from the bench, and looked on in horror as the other team rallied in the sixth and final inning to win the game 5-4. I cried because we lost, but I took solace in the fact that I was not the losing pitcher of record.

If I had been out there and given up the winning run, I'm not sure I would have survived it. My world would have come crashing down. But it wasn't my fault. I wasn't the losing pitcher.

I didn't lose the game.

The next morning, I was on the couch at home watching cartoons, when my old man walked into the room, standing in the doorway that led to the bedrooms and bathrooms. We were talking about the game, when he said the worst thing he possibly could have said:

"Well, if our best pitcher hadn't been throwing curveballs all night, we wouldn't have lost the game."

I felt like I had been run over by a truck.

My dad, the one person in the world I most wanted and could never get approval from, was blaming me for the loss. How could he say that? I was absolutely and completed destroyed.

I played two more years of baseball and made two more all-star teams, two more years of football, ran track and played basketball in junior high, but by my sophomore year in high school, I'd had enough.

Whatever relationship I had with my dad was in shambles. My anger had grown from a simmer to a boil over those two years, and there was constant conflict in our house. It was pretty much a war zone, at times.

He asked me once when we were battling over something if I wanted to go out in the backyard and fight. I was 140 pounds at best, while he weighed in at about 250. I just laughed.

Quitting sports was a major turning point in my life. Suddenly, I no longer had any identity. Remember, I measured my self-worth on my sports accomplishments. My friends were all athletes. My life revolved around sports. Now, there was nothing. I was nothing. Who was I?

I still hung out at first with my jock friends, but it wasn't the same. I really didn't belong anymore. For about a year, I was lost at sea. This could have been when some depression started kicking in. I'm not really sure.

Then one day, I discovered marijuana, and it was like I had found the answer. Not only did it feel really good to get high, I gained instant membership to a very popular crowd – the freaks. The wild and crazy kids who hung out in front of the school every morning, smoking pot and cigarettes, giving all the teachers and principals a hard time all day, skipping classes to go play foosball down at the corner store, going out with a bunch of hot, loose girls. Just generally having a great time.

I belonged somewhere again. Found a new identity. Just like that. And like everything else, I went at it with full intensity. Grew my hair long and smoked pot every day, drank a little, graduated to pills and powders, rebelling at anything that even resembled an authority figure.

For the next fifteen years, that's what I lived for – getting high.

Chapter Three

Some of the risk factors for developing depression include such things as traumatic or long-term stressful situations; difficult personal relationships; low self-esteem; pessimism; being overly self-critical; alcohol and drug abuse; history of depression, alcoholism, suicide in the family.

Um, check. Check, check. Check, check, check.

Not only were some of those factors in play for me, they ALL were. Every single one of them. My entire childhood was stressful. Granted, a lot of it was self-imposed due to my extreme perfectionist personality – along with never knowing when an explosion of sorts was going to rock the house – but it was stressful, nonetheless.

My relationship with my father was difficult, at best. Self-esteem was non-existent. I inherited his negative attitude about everything, was extremely self-critical, had major insecurity, was drinking and drugging to excess on a regular basis, and coming from a family full of mental illness.

I was a shipwreck waiting to happen.

As soon as I graduated from high school, I moved into a friend's apartment, bummed around for a month or two, then went to work for Brown & Root, Inc. as an office runner, ferrying mail and messages and such between their various offices around town. This was way before the age of computers. My old man worked for the massive engineering company, as well, repairing printing equipment in their various shops. This put him in contact with engineers and project managers and the like, and at some point he learned about an opening for an entry-level drafting job that included on-the-job training.

Long story short, he got me an interview and I got that job, enjoyed it, and worked my way up to senior electrical draftsman by the time I was twenty-three years old. I was fast, neat, accurate and good at the job. My perfectionism came in handy.

I also got married two months before I turned 19. I won't say it was a mistake, because a wonderful daughter came out of that twelve-year union, but I didn't really want to get married. I tried to back out once, but felt too much guilt when my future bride cried and pitched a fit and threatened to kill herself, so I went ahead and did it, anyway.

I wasn't a terrible husband, but not a very good one, either. We lived a partying lifestyle, and I went to work most of the time, paid my bills and all that good stuff. But I was far from a loving, attentive husband, in the traditional sense. We were two kids playing house, basically, and of course it did not end well.

When I told my supervisor at work, a guy named Mike from Ocala, Florida, who was in his mid-30s, that I was getting married, he looked at me incredulously and said, "What for?" I don't remember my response, but his response to my response was this:

"Let me tell you something. When you turn twenty-five or twenty-six, things are going to change. It's going to be like flipping a light switch. You're not going to think the same way; you're going to be a different person. C'mon, man, you don't want to get married."

Of course, I knew better. Why should I listen to someone fifteen years older, who has been there and done that? As it turned out, ol' Mike was exactly right.

More on that later.

After about three years of marriage, a number of our friends started having babies, and my wife started hounding me about having one, too. I put her off for a while, and then – without any meaningful discussion, planning, or consideration of the long-term implications of such a life-changing decision – I told her on the phone one day at work, "Okay, let's do it."

And so we did.

One windy February day the following year, my first child was born. I remember my wife waiting until I woke up that morning, and telling me, "I think it's time."

Me being the kind, gentle, supportive husband, my response was: "What do you mean, you *think* it's time? Is it, or isn't it?"

"I don't know," she said, tearfully.

Nice.

So I called work and told the boss I would not be in; we packed up and headed to the hospital, and sure enough, it was time. It took forever, but eventually, there I was, in the delivery room, watching a baby being born. My baby. As they cleaned her up and looked her over, the doctor suddenly said, "Uh-oh."

The room immediately got quiet.

Two people you never want to hear say, "Uh-oh," are a dentist and a doctor.

There was a marked cloudiness, large white spots, on the surface of both her little eyes, one quite a bit worse than the other. A normal healthy baby, otherwise, but the eye thing was something nobody had never seen before. They had no idea what might have caused it. The only thing they knew is that it was not good.

I was beside myself – as usual, my first reaction was mostly all about me – and I asked my mother out in the hallway, "What if she's blind? What are we gonna do?"

Mama put her arm around my shoulders and said gently, "Don't borrow trouble, son."

Good advice. Too bad I had no idea what it meant.

A short time later, a nurse came and asked me if I would like to see my baby. Since they did not know what kind of strange affliction might have caused the opaqueness on her eyes, Stacy was isolated from the rest of the babies in the nursery. I followed the nurse down and around to a back door, and sat in a white, wooden rocking chair next to the wall.

Someone else handed me this little warm bundle, tightly wrapped in a pink blanket with light blue stripes, and as soon as I held her close, I felt a surge of energy travel up my arms and straight into my heart. It was strong and it was real. I literally felt love, or heaven, or God, or something, coming out of that little newborn baby.

I never felt anything like that before or since. Talk about instant bonding. I was hopelessly head over heels.

Because of the eye condition, they let us take her the next day to a specialist, who examined her and took what seemed like gallons of blood out of her tiny arm, poking and jabbing and sticking. At one point, I was about to step in and say, "That's enough," but the doctor

17

apparently sensed my growing anxiety and said, "It's okay, dad, we're almost done."

Turned out that Stacy had some fairly rare condition that somehow caused her corneas to adhere to the rest of the eye, instead of being convex-shaped, like a contact lens. That was it. No sinister underlying disease causing the problem.

One eye was considerably worse than the other, but the specialist said she would definitely not be blind, and the prescribed treatment was amazingly simple.

We had to put drops in her eyes every day to dilate them, with the idea being that the action of the pupil expanding and contracting would loosen the corneal adhesions. She had to wear a little eye patch over her less-affected eye, to try and strengthen the one that would be weaker, the one with more adhesions, and she was fitted with a miniature set of pink, plastic eyeglasses, mostly to protect the "good eye."

So, all was well, and Stacy turned out just fine. Life went on as usual, without much change in our habits, except now we took a kid with us when we went to visit friends and "party." We stayed home more in the beginning, but as Stacy got a little older, we went back to our normal lifestyle, filled with rock and roll, cases of Lone Star longnecks, bags of weed, and other assorted substances.

By the time I reached twenty-five or twenty-six – exactly as Mike had predicted – I was becoming more and more unhappy. I was tired of being tied down; tired of the responsibility; tired of going to work; tired of paying bills; lamenting everything I imagined I had missed out on by getting married so young.

I was still working at Brown and Root, but my partying habits had gotten out of control. I remember going to work quite often with massive hangovers – the kind where even your eyeballs hurt. This was in the early 1980s, and the company was undergoing massive layoffs because of the oil crunch, and I became a victim of the personnel cutbacks.

Actually, I was not a victim at all. I was one of the best draftsmen in the division, received annual promotions and pay increases, and was not a target for layoffs, as far as I knew. But I decided that I *wanted* to lose my job and go on unemployment. So I basically quit working, stopped producing like I always had, and turned myself from an asset into a liability.

One day, my supervisor – not Mike; another guy from the Philippines whose name has long since been forgotten – called me into his cubicle and asked if everything was okay. Is something wrong, he wondered, with a look of genuine concern on his face.

This was my brilliant response.

"No, I just want to be laid off. Why don't you give my job to somebody who wants it?"

The guy looked at me in disbelief. People were being sent packing every Friday, and everybody was living in fear of a visit from the project manager. Here was some young knucklehead asking to have his job taken away?

"Okay," he said, shrugging his shoulders, and I went back to my drafting table.

A few days later, after I came back from a break, there was a note stuck on my table saying the big boss wanted to see me in his office.

My heart started pounding in my chest. Oh, shit, what the hell have I done?

I went up there and he sat me down and gave me the whole, "We're very sorry, but we're cutting back, and you're being laid off," spiel, and that was it. Next Friday, I was one of the ones carrying a cardboard box out the door at quitting time.

Chapter Four

According to a survey conducted by the Centers for Disease Control and Prevention, approximately nine percent of Americans report being depressed once in a while, and 3.4 percent suffer from major depression.

That's somewhere between eleven million and twenty-eight million people.

The World Health Organization, meanwhile, calls depression "the leading cause of disability worldwide," and "a major contributor to the overall global burden of disease," affecting as many as three hundred-fifty million people of all ages.

Clearly, this is not an uncommon condition.

There are a lot of struggling people out there. And here's one thing I have learned, that I can confidently pass along as an absolute, indisputable truth of life:

If you think nobody knows how you feel – you are wrong.

Somebody, somewhere, knows how you feel. In fact, a lot of people know how you feel. More than you could ever imagine.

Trust me. It is absolutely true.

So there I was, out of a job for the first time since I was sixteen years old, and filing for unemployment compensation. I also told my wife I was moving out, leaving her and my five-year-old daughter to basically fend for themselves.

It is a little hazy now – that was thirty years ago – and I honestly don't remember how she took it, but I packed some clothes and headed across town to my grandmother's house, and mostly hung out every day with some other derelict friends at a nearby apartment complex and got loaded every day for the next six months.

When the unemployment benefits started to run out, I went back home and announced that I was going to enroll full-time at San Jacinto Junior College, where I went for a year while working as a security guard downtown before transferring to the University of Houston.

I had always planned to go to college when I was a kid, and working for Brown & Root all those years reinforced that idea even more. I worked five-and-a-half days a week alongside electrical engineers who were all around my age, maybe a little older, but no different than me, no smarter. The only thing they had that I didn't was a college degree.

So I went back to school, and decided to study journalism. I wanted to be a sports reporter. That day my old man came over to the apartment to give me a check for the first semester's tuition – he said he always told me he'd do what he could to help with college, and wanted to keep his promise – he asked what I was going to study. When I told him I was going to be a sports reporter, I thought he'd be pretty excited, since he was also a huge sports nut.

Wrong.

After I told him, there was nothing but an awkward silence. He did not say a word. It was more than a little uncomfortable.

But that was my plan. That's what I wanted to do, and that's what I did.

I had a great time going to college, commuting across town every day to the campus via two city buses. One bus went from near our apartment to downtown, where I got off and transferred to another bus going to UH. Same thing in reverse to get back home.

For the first time in a long time, I felt like I was really accomplishing something, and I have always enjoyed reading, studying and learning.

I pretty quickly got a gig with the campus newspaper, and then a professor recommended me for a reporting job with a neighborhood weekly in nearby West University Place. Sometime after that, another professor told me about an opening with a publication called Golfer Magazines, which had offices along the Katy Freeway. I went over there one day, interviewed with the owner, a well-known Houston area publisher named Bob Gray Sr., and got a job as a part-time writer and photographer.

All this time, I was working hard, getting good grades, earning a variety of academic scholarships, and also cultivating an alcohol habit that was growing more and more serious.

On my way home each day from UH, I developed an ingenious system for catching a nice after-school buzz.

When I got off the first bus downtown, I'd walk down the street and buy a forty-ounce bottle of malt liquor, sit and drink that while I waited for my transfer bus. Then, instead of riding all the way home, I'd get off about halfway, outside a convenience store, pick up another forty-ouncer, and suck that down before the next bus came along.

At one point, I even befriended a guy at school who had a prescription for these big, blue valium, and he'd give me one to take on the way home, as well. So by the time I got there, I was feeling pretty darned good.

Nevertheless, when I graduated, I quickly got an offer for a reporting job with the newspaper in Richardson, Texas, a suburb of Dallas. I accepted right away, and I remember making the announcement during a Christmas gathering at my mother's house.

It was another one of those awkward moments, and not what I was expecting. No congratulations, or "That's great!", or anything like that. Mostly, a bunch of sideways glances around the room, since I was going to move up there from Houston by myself. My wife and daughter would stay behind, since I expected it to be a temporary gig. I knew in the newspaper business, the way to move up is to move around, work for a while in a place, gain some experience; then head to a larger market.

Apparently, the family did not think it was such a great idea.

And, really, it wasn't.

In fact, it was probably the beginning of the end of the marriage. It took another year for things to completely dissolve, but dissolve they did.

I worked for the Richardson Daily News for a few months, and really enjoyed it, but I was lonely living up there alone, in an apartment by Fair Park, staying to myself and drinking a lot.

One of my first days at work, as it neared time to go home, a girl named Elizabeth told me she and some of the other reporters were going out for Chinese food later and would I like to join them? Like an idiot, I said, no thanks, and that was the last invitation I ever received.

Why did I turn it down?

Easy.

I figured going out to dinner would cut too much into my all-important drinking time. So I did my usual thing of stopping by a store on the way home and buying a twelve-pack of beer and a frozen TV dinner. Sat in the apartment by myself watching TV and getting hammered.

Eventually, there was a family emergency back home in Houston, and I pretty much used that as an excuse to move back. I told my editor that something had happened and I was leaving, threw my shit in the car and took off. The apartment complex came after me for breaking my lease, as did the furniture store where I had rented a sofa-sleeper, but I just blew them off, as well.

The reunion with my little family was short-lived, as my wife asked me to leave a few months after I came back. I did not know it at the time, but she had already fallen for someone else, a guy who just so happened to be an old friend to us both, a member of the old party scene that we both frequented for years and years.

I never saw that coming – maybe if I'd been more sober more often – even though the wife had been trying to tell me for some time that "our marriage is in trouble."

I put up a fuss for a while – begged, pleaded, and cried quite a bit, mostly over losing my number one enabler – but in the end, I went and moved in with a divorced friend and her pre-teen son, who just so happened to live in the neighborhood where I grew up.

By that time, I was a bit of a mess: abusing alcohol on a regular basis, delivering sandwiches for a delicatessen by day, and working for the now-defunct Houston Post at night, helping edit copy and put together the sports section.

Then one day I got a call from one of my old journalism professors, telling me about a job with a newspaper called the Temple Daily Telegram. I had never heard of the paper, or the city of Temple, except that it was some little podunk place in the middle of nowhere, so I balked at the idea of going there.

My professor said, 'Well, do you want to keep working part-time for the Post, or do you want to be a full-time reporter?'

Of course, that made a lot of sense, so I called the managing editor in Temple and he basically offered me the job over the phone. I drove up there for an interview, looked around for an apartment, and went to work a short time later.

Chapter Five

According to the Office on Women's Health, U.S. Department of Health and Human Services, more women than men are likely to be diagnosed with depression in any given year. Part of the reason for that, experts say, is that men are less likely to recognize or acknowledge symptoms of depression, which once was thought of as a women's disease linked to hormones and PMS (premenstrual syndrome).

This obviously stereotypical viewpoint is still around, and could explain why many men are reluctant to seek appropriate treatment.

The symptoms of clinical depression are similar in both men and women, although female sufferers tend to be more sad and emotional, while males may be more irritable, aggressive, and even hostile.

For me, I had no clue about depression, and for a long time, did not really believe it was a "disease" that needed treatment. I always thought of depression as a kind of cop-out. Sometimes you feel good; sometimes you feel bad. Such is life. Get over it.

After my parents got divorced, when I was in my early twenties, my father went into a major tailspin and did not come out of it for years and years. I did not have much to do with him during all that, because I thought it was a bunch of bullshit, basically. I thought he was just feeling sorry for himself, and looking for sympathy. I sure wasn't going to give him any of that, because I thought he was pretty much getting what he deserved.

Like father, like son, he was a pretty shitty husband.

Someone told me they went out to see him in that ramshackle old house he had moved out to the country and never fixed up, and he was sitting there moping, surrounded by tall stacks of empty pizza boxes and other garbage and clutter.

I didn't feel sorry for him. In my mind, he had brought it all upon himself. Tough shit.

When I moved to Temple for my new job, everything I owned fit inside an old red Chevrolet Cavalier that I eventually drove into the ground. It really is important, apparently, to change the oil in a car once in a while. I had some clothes, a few dishes, some forks and spoons, a portable black-and-white television set with rabbit ear antenna, two sleeping bags, a pillow, and that was about it.

For three months, I lived on the floor of the little apartment I rented for $150 a month, I think it was. I went to work, did my thing, and then came home and ate TV dinners, 7-Eleven hot dogs, and drank myself into unconsciousness.

One of the first things I had to do after I moved was to go check in at the county adult probation offices, since I was serving a two-year probation for driving under the influence back in Houston.

Here are the gory details surrounding that incident:

This was after I moved back to Houston from Richardson, and the wife and I were visiting her mother, sitting around talking and drinking – them talking and me mostly drinking – when I decided that downing nearly a fifth of Scotch by myself wasn't enough, so I hopped in the car and drove down to the corner convenience store for a six-pack and some cigarettes.

I never made it back to the house.

About halfway home, flashing lights suddenly appeared in my rearview mirror. I panicked, hit the gas and took off. All I could think about was getting back to our apartment, which was just outside the neighborhood where we were visiting mom-in-law.

I went about a half-mile down FM 1960, whipped into the apartment complex parking lot – nearly hitting several parked cars in the process, they told me later – and stopped in a space just outside our front door. As I got out of the car and shut the door, a none-too-pleased deputy sheriff grabbed me, turned me around, tossed me up against the trunk, and slapped handcuffs on me.

I was pretty out of it, mouthing off, giving the guy a hard time, when he finally got me to a substation not far from there, where he allowed me to make a phone call. I tried to call the wife, but unfortunately, no one answered the phone and I wound up going downtown, to the notorious Harris County Jail.

They kept me for a while in a holding cell at the substation, and I was still raising hell, banging on the bars, demanding to go to the bathroom and I don't remember what all. At some point, I unzipped my pants and flooded half the cell with piss. When the deputy came in to get me, he saw what I had done and slammed me up against the far brick wall.

"You're going downtown," he snarled, his face close to mine.

That scared the hell out of me.

When I got there in the wee morning hours, after they searched me and some other new arrivals, we were all lined up for booking. My turn came, and the jailer was asking me questions and filling out paperwork, then he told me to place my right thumb print on a card or some sort of document. I misunderstood and printed the wrong thumb, and he said, "Your right thumb, dumbass," or something like that.

I didn't say anything, but I gave him a very easy-to-interpret "fuck you" look, and he immediately stood up, came around the counter, grabbed hold of me and started marching me down the hall. *Oh, shit*, I thought, *what now?*

He took me a ways down some corridor, stopped in front of a metal door, told me not to move, took out his keys, unlocked the door, and shoved me inside. It was a small, dirty cell, and there were two rough-looking dudes already inside, one sitting on a bench with his head down, and the other on the floor, curled around a toilet.

I thought for sure I was going to get my ass kicked. I figured that was why the deputy put me in there.

Nothing unusual happened, though, and after a while, those two guys were taken somewhere else, leaving me in there alone, until the door opened and a little short jailer told me to step outside. I did so and waited by the door, as instructed, while he went back inside and took a long, slow piss, then – without flushing the toilet – told me to get back inside. He said something about me flooding the cell back at the substation, so this was supposed to be some kind of payback, I guess, and then he slammed the door shut.

I sat down on the bench, reached over and flushed away the stench.

Eventually, they put me in a big drunk tank, which was full of all kinds of scary-looking characters. There was a phone in there that allowed collect calls, and I tried to get a hold of my wife again, and this time she answered.

"Where are you?" she asked.

"In jail."

"Where?"

"I don't know," I said. "Can you come get me out?"

Sometime in the mid-morning hours the next day, I heard my name being called, and I was being released.

I walked out into the sunshine in downtown Houston, my left wrist so swollen from fighting against the handcuffs that I could not put my watch back on, and my wife came along and picked me up and took me home, where I proceeded to get good and sloshed.

My mother-in-law had an attorney friend and he agreed to take my case for $500, but I was doomed from the start, despite the fact that I had refused a breathalyzer test after I got arrested.

The first time we met with an assistant district attorney, he showed video from that night at the jail and there was no challenging what we saw on that black-and-white tape.

I was standing barefoot in some little room, with a camera mounted high on the wall in one corner, hands in my pants pockets, swaying back and forth just slightly, as the officer asked me several times about taking a breathalyzer.

Things didn't look too bad at that point.

Then, when it was time to leave the room, I turned around, immediately lost my balance and slammed hard up against the wall to my left, falling completely out of camera range.

My attorney looked at me, with sort of a wry smile, and said, "Well, John, you were doing pretty good until right there at the end."

He and the ADA both laughed.

I did not think it was real funny.

So I wound up pleading nolo contendre, got put on probation, and ordered to undergo some alcohol classes. When we got outside the courthouse, my attorney shook my hand before we parted ways and warned me, "If they catch you again, they'll put you *under* the jail."

Whatever.

The only thing that changed after that was I started wearing my seat belt when I drove. I always had a beer in between my legs – usually a quart bottle – and I figured that if I got pulled over for not wearing a seat belt, I'd be in big trouble. So after that, I always buckled up.

For some reason, I was completely honest when I went later for a court-ordered evaluation that involved answering a whole slew of questions about drinking habits, and they labeled me a chronic alcoholic. The first time I reported to a probation officer, he ordered me to attend two AA meetings a week.

Again, whatever.

That was in January, and I never went. Around the middle of February, I moved to Temple.

Chapter Six

Depression often begins at a young age – the teen years, twenties, thirties – but it can creep up and grab hold at any time.

I am sure I was depressed many moons before I finally recognized or admitted it, or even suspected it. When you are used to swimming in sewage all the time, you tend to get used to the smell.

Serious depression, again, is a lot different from feeling sad or bummed out because you lost a bet on the Super Bowl; your boyfriend or girlfriend dumped you; your wife or husband left and wants a divorce; you lost your job; wrecked your car; some mean person hurt your feelings.

The most common symptom of true depression is a hopeless or helpless outlook on life. You are no longer in control. Nothing matters any more. Who cares? What difference does it make? Nobody cares about my problems. Nobody cares if I live or die. What is the point of going on? I'm tired of living.

At the time I got arrested, I was working as a telephone bill collector for one of those fly-by-night companies that harasses people with overdue and unpaid credit card balances. Actually, I only worked there for a month, because my heart really wasn't into badgering people on the phone to send me money or else, so then it was on to The Container Store, near The Galleria shopping center on Westheimer.

I did okay at that job for a while, sort of enjoyed it, but eventually I got fired after failing to show up for my scheduled shift several times in a row. I blamed it on reading the schedule wrong, but it was really due to irresponsibility and alcohol.

When I got canned from that job, it was pretty much the last straw for my wife.

We were living in that apartment near the subdivision on FM 1960 where I got busted, and one day in October, she told me it was over. I cried and begged and pleaded, more than once, but what I didn't yet know is that it was over – she was already involved with that other guy.

To get away from me and my drinking, she was taking our daughter on the weekends to visit her brother – my former best friend – in Austin. They would spend the weekend there, while I stayed home and drank myself silly. During these visits, she got involved with a dude we both had known for years and years. He always had a thing for her, and now, he saw his opportunity, and swept in.

I spent the next three or four months working as a lunchtime delivery driver for the deli, and nights at the Houston Post. I visited my daughter some on weekends, usually taking her with me to spend the night at my grandmother's house. The place I was staying was not exactly suitable for kids.

Then, I got the job in Temple and off I went.

During the three-hour drive from Houston, I had to stop at a rest area alongside the highway and sleep for a while, since I had stayed up half the night before getting loaded. I finally got to town shortly before I was to report to work, stopped by an Albertson's grocery store to get a pair of socks and a razor, put on my socks and shoes and shaved in the car, then headed to my new job.

For the next few months, I covered the general assignment beat in and around Temple, settling in to the job, getting to know the system and my co-workers, who were all very nice. On guy, in particular, by the name of Max, lived in the same apartment complex where I wound up, and so we hung out some. Mostly, though, I kept to myself, drinking a lot and driving back to Houston on the weekends to see my daughter and a girl I had met shortly before the move, while delivering a lunch order to her office.

I was hanging on by a thread at this point, doing a decent enough job, then going home to drink by myself, laying on my sleeping bag and watching TV.

What I did not know it at the time, but found out about six months later, was that my new boss was keeping an eye on me, after getting at least one phone call asking about the reporter he sent to cover some event. The guy reeked of alcohol, whoever it was said. Steve, the paper's managing editor, asked Max if I had a drinking problem. Max lied and told him he had no idea, even though he himself struggled with alcohol abuse and recognized pretty quickly what was going on with me.

And although I was on probation, I continued to drink and drive. I drank a beer or two for breakfast, had beer for lunch, beer for dinner, with maybe a convenience store hot dog or a TV dinner. Any time I left the office to go cover a story, I stopped and bought a beer, then popped a peppermint in my mouth and thought nobody would be the wiser.

It sounds incredible, but I was drinking about a case a day of whatever I could find that was on sale. It didn't matter what it tasted like. I was after the effect, not the enjoyment.

Things came to a head three months later, toward the end of May 1989, when I woke up after a three-day weekend of heavy drinking. I was so sick that I could not even swallow water. It came right back up.

Since arriving in Temple and checking in with the county probation office there, I had been going to Alcoholics Anonymous meetings twice a week, which was a requirement of my probation. I had to get this little card signed by whoever was chairing the meeting, and then present it each month to my probation officer.

I didn't want to go to those meetings any more then than I did back in Houston, but the first time I met with the new probation officer, he asked me if I had been going to my meetings. I said, no, and he looked at me over his reading glasses and said, "Why not?"

I don't remember what I answered, but I remember what he said next.

"You wanna get locked up?"

He handed me a card and told me about these noon "brown bag" meetings at some place on 23rd Street, and told me I could go to those.

Shit, I thought, this old redneck is going to throw my ass in jail, if I don't go. So I went to a meeting the next day on my lunch break.

When I pulled up in front of the place, it was an old frame house with peeling paint, and big wooden steps leading up to a rotting porch with a big hole you had to walk around to get to the front door.

There was a long conference-type table in the front room, and you could see through into the kitchen, where people were coming in and out with cups of coffee. Folding chairs lined the walls all around the table, and I sat in one of those near the front door.

It was pretty interesting to hear everyone talk about their drinking adventures and misadventures – one guy who would later become my first sponsor had seven DWIs – although I drank before and after the meetings, and had no intention of stopping.

One thing that got my attention, though, was the stories people told about their feelings. The reasons why they were miserable, and why they drank too much. These were people from all walks of life: businessmen wearing coats and ties; housewives; burly bikers riding Harleys; old, retired guys with missing teeth; young mechanics and factory workers; pretty young girls; farmers; truck drivers; teachers; lawyers; doctors.

Listening to this diverse group of folks talk at meetings, I realized something I never knew before – other people felt the same way I did. Had gone through a lot of the same things I did.

Let me say that again, because it's important.

I realized for the first time in my life, a college-educated 32-year-old man, that I was not unique. Other people in the world – a lot of them – dealt with the same hurts, fears, disappointments, regrets that I had experienced all my life.

I never knew that. I thought I was the only one. That was pretty cool to learn, and it made a pretty big impression on me, but I wasn't ready to give up my alcohol.

Didn't need to. I could stop drinking if I wanted to – I just didn't want to. That's what I told myself.

Then came that Monday, after the massive three-day bender. I was so sick, and I was tired of being sick all the time. I decided to go to a meeting that night, even though I didn't have to go to fulfill my weekly quota of meetings.

I walked into that old house on 23rd Street with the rickety stairs and the huge hole in the front porch, and when the meeting began and introductions went around the room, I said for the first time, "I'm John, and I'm an alcoholic." Prior to that, I'd always simply said, "I'm John."

After the meeting, I went home, walked into my bedroom and knelt beside my newly purchased used water bed. I clasped my hands together, bowed my head, and asked God to help me.

My prayer went something like this:

"God, if you're out there, please help me stop drinking and stop being so unhappy. I can't do it by myself. Amen."

That was about it.

Then I got up, walked into the living room and picked up a book I'd checked out a few days earlier from the downtown library. I don't remember the title, but it was a story written by a former *New York Times* reporter about her recovery from alcohol addiction through AA.

I was browsing the library shelves one day, walking up and down looking at titles, when that one practically jumped out at me.

So I grabbed the book and sat down on my fifty-dollar thrift store couch, and started reading. I don't remember exactly any more, but when I came across a passage in which the author was talking about her selfishness being one of the roots of her problems – as soon as I read that word, selfish – something strange happened.

Chapter Seven

When I finally figured out in my mid-40s that maybe I was depressed and decided to try and get some help, I made an appointment with a local hospital mental health center, underwent some extensive evaluations, and was officially diagnosed not only with depression, but with anxiety, to boot.

According to the Anxiety and Depression Association of America, around half of people diagnosed with depression also suffer from anxiety. Many symptoms are similar, although with depression, a person usually dwells about negative things from the past that make the future seem bleak, while anxiety focuses irrationally on things that have not yet happened.

Anxiety can include such things as getting sick to your stomach, heart palpitations, headaches and gastrointestinal disturbances. People who are depressed have little to no energy and drive, lack motivation to get up and go about their normal daily activities.

Experts say that anxiety can often come before the onset of depression. People who are anxious in childhood have an increased chance of becoming depressed later in life.

Some believe that such conditions are a combination of nature and nurture: some personality traits are passed along in our genetic material from our parents, and some are picked up along the way from friends, family members and our living environment.

For me, that sounds about right.

Depression runs in my family. I was anxious as a child, constantly looking for love, affection and approval, a feeling of safety and security.

It is an odd thing, but even today, I have a lot of trouble sleeping. I had an overnight sleep study done a number of years ago after I started nodding off behind the wheel as I drove home from work, and it revealed that at least part of my problem was severe restless leg syndrome throughout the night, keeping me from achieving a full, restful quality of sleep.

Along with that, though, is also an underlying anxiety of some sort that makes it hard for me to relax and fall asleep. The slightest sound can wake me up, even bring my head snapping up off the pillow. It is like I'm afraid to fall deeply asleep, to be too vulnerable.

There is nothing in my past that would have caused something like this; nothing I can remember, anyway.

Just another sign of a troubled mind, I suppose.

But back to the story …

When I read the word "selfish" in that book, the room suddenly became sort of blurry, hazy, out of focus. Time seemed to slow way down, and I lowered the book and kind of slumped back into the couch.

As I sat there, in sort of a trance, what felt like a large hand came and rested gently on top of my head, and what I have always described as these "large, twisted knots of pain and confusion" started being pulled up and out of the top of my head, from deep inside me. I could actually feel a physical sensation of something like a knotted rope that kept coming and coming, up and out of my body.

It took what seemed like a long time, and when it was over, the fuzzy surroundings disappeared, my sense of time and space returned to normal, and I felt completely relaxed.

Most importantly, somehow I knew everything was going to be all right. I was going to be okay. I did not hear an audible voice or anything like that, but something told me very clearly, in my head and my heart, that everything was going to be all right now.

It was a miracle.

The next morning, I got up to go to work, and was standing in my kitchen, leaning against the counter, drinking a cup of coffee, when it suddenly occurred to me – hey, I didn't drink last night, did I?

I actually had to stop and think about it for a few seconds.

It was the first time in years that I had gone that long without alcohol.

That night, or maybe the next night, after another AA meeting, I walked down to the corner store and bought a twelve-pack of Sprite. Not cheap beer or a gallon of wine, but soft drinks. As I headed back home, through the apartment complex across the street,

I looked up at the star-filled sky and thought, "How weird is this? I'm walking home from the store, completely sober, carrying a twelve-pack of soda ..."

After that, I spent the majority of my spare time either at AA meetings, or hanging around with other AA members. I was high on life, and enjoying it for the first time in a long, long time.

For maybe the first time ever, I was starting to understand things about myself, and feeling like I belonged in the world.

At meetings, people always talked about what a struggle it was to not drink, one day at a time, and all that. People talked about relapsing, going back out and getting drunk. For me, there was no struggle. Some way, somehow, the urge to drink was completely gone.

Prior to the miracle, I was either drinking, thinking about drinking, or on my way to get something to drink. All the time. Every day. It was the way I lived. The way I survived.

Now, nothing. No struggles; no fighting.

I did not drink, and I was happy about it. I did not miss it at all.

It was truly an amazing thing.

My friend, Max, from work, who was one of those in and out of sobriety, introduced me to a friend of his girlfriend, and we hit it off right away and started seeing each other regularly. She had a kid and I know she was looking for a husband, but I was not ready for that, so – even though she was a wonderful woman who treated me wonderfully and probably would have made a great wife – after a few months, I sort of dumped her.

It was not my finest moment, especially when she came knocking at my door one Saturday morning with a rose in one hand and a letter in the other, and I had to tell her that now was not a good time for a visit.

I didn't tell her there was another woman in my bed at the time, but I could tell by the look on her face that she knew.

That second sober relationship lasted about a year-and-a-half, but this girl was a lot younger and I decided early on that the long-term possibilities were not good. Even though she begged me at one point, "Please, just let me love you," I never wanted to feel the agony of a broken heart that I felt back in Houston when my wife sent me packing.

The truth is, I told myself shortly after we got together that I was going to break up with her before she could break up with me. I had been devastated by my divorce, and I never wanted to feel that kind of pain ever again.

So, that relationship ended, and I was single for a while. Then, my mother came to see me one weekend when my ten-year-old daughter was also in town for a visit, and we all went to dinner at a steak house in Temple.

I was lonely for female companionship, our waitress was friendly and attractive, and I noticed she was not wearing a ring, so I left a note with my name and phone number on our order ticket when we left. A few days later, she called and we decided to go out.

That was the beginning of two of the worst years of my life. This woman turned out to be a complete psycho, a master manipulator, sociopath, and user of men who no doubt spotted me coming a mile away. I am sure it took her all of five minutes talking to me before she knew she had found an easy mark.

Chapter Eight

According to a number of scientific studies, both nature and nurture play a role in whether or not someone develops depression.

Most experts agree that there is no single cause. Instead, it is more widely believed that a combination of factors help trigger the sometimes crippling disorder, including such things as brain chemistry, genetics, hormonal imbalances, and environment.

Some research indicates that people with a "first-degree relative" who suffers depression (parent or sibling) are three times more likely to follow suit. Other studies say not true, and that such a finding discounts self-determination – the ability for people to overcome and control their own destiny, thought patterns, attitudes, and outlooks.

In other words, genetic factors are not a trap from which there is no escape.

A child who grows up with someone suffering from depression may be more susceptible to developing depression, but it may be more a matter of mimicking the behavior they witness and experience than some sort of biologically caused condition.

Nature versus nurture.

In many cases, depression can be brought on by major life events, such as a loved one's death, serious health problems, unemployment; divorce.

And, again, depression is not the same as feeling sad. True depression often lasts for months or years. Relationships often fail. A person may become unable to work.

So, I met this waitress, and we went dancing one night at a local country and western club. She told me she had three kids, and that kind of startled me, but she was charming my pants off – literally – and I fell hook, line and sinker.

For a while, things were going okay. I gave up my apartment, and moved in with her and the kids, but one night shortly after that she did not come home from work.

She did not come home until the next afternoon.

When her ten-year-old daughter got up in the morning and walked into the living room, rubbing her eyes and asking, 'Where's mom?', I expected some sort of surprised reaction when I told her I had no idea, that she had been out all night and not come home, but she just yawned, and said, 'Oh.'

Apparently, this was not unusual behavior.

I really don't want to go back and re-hash the whole incredible experience, but I will say this woman very nearly destroyed me, before it was all over. Almost as soon as this new relationship began, it was a disaster.

When we met, I had been clean and sober for about two years, and I was really naïve. I had never known a true sociopath, and I honestly did not realize that people were capable of just blatantly using other people, looking you in the eye and telling lies over and over and over, with no regard whatsoever to how much pain they inflicted in the process. Convincing you that everything was your fault. On, and on, and on.

I was desperate to be loved – as I had been all my life – not fond of being alone, and also experiencing what I considered a second chance at life, in which God or somebody had loved me enough to save me from myself, and now I had met someone who I thought could use the same chance. Obviously this woman had baggage, but I thought that if I loved her enough, all the old wounds would heal and everything would be great.

What an idiot.

I got a part-time gig as a photographer's assistant around this time, and he asked me one day, as we were discussing my miserable situation: "So, when are you going to get rid of your white horse?"

Getting involved with this crazy woman was definitely not one of my better moves – and it took some caring friends from AA to wake me up and convince me to leave, which I eventually did – but I think we were brought together for a reason.

The reason this psycho and I were brought together, (and) the reason I suffered two solid years of absolute torment and abuse, was so that my youngest daughter could be born. That is the only possible reason. She, too, suffered at the hands of this deeply troubled woman, with whom she lived up until her senior year in high school – and that is one of my lasting regrets, that I didn't take her to live with me – but my daughter is a special person who I think is going to do something extraordinary in her life.

I never went after custody because I thought taking my daughter away would do more harm than good – quite possibly causing World War III to erupt. This woman had talked about cutting people's throats, and dumping bodies in abandoned water wells out in the country. I had no idea what she was really capable of doing.

When my daughter spent weekends with me, her mother was constantly calling, supposedly to check on her and make sure she was all right.

My daughter told me one day several years ago, as we were riding in my car, that she was "scared to death" of me most of her life. Why? That was easy to figure out. Because her mother was constantly poisoning her mind. She is the type of evil person who would not come right out and say things, but I can imagine conversations like this: "Now, if he touches you, or tries to hurt you, or anything like that, I will come and get you, okay?"

Putting ideas into the poor kid's head.

Pure evil.

When I finally got out of there, I was homeless, broke, and once again, everything I owned fit in my car. Back to square one.

I moved in with a friend for a while, until a local television reporter I knew who owned a small trailer park fixed me up with a rundown, little two-bedroom mobile home that was nice and cheap. I got a roommate pretty quickly, a fellow AA member serving in the Army just down the road at Fort Hood, and so it was plenty affordable.

Thus began yet another life rebuilding process.

Chapter Nine

Emotional or physical trauma, grief, financial problems and unemployment are a few examples of well-known depression triggers, but there are plenty more causes.

Some other factors in the onset of depression include such things as:

Smoking – while people who are prone to depression may be more likely to pick up the habit, nicotine is also said to affect neurotransmitter activity in the brain, leading to higher levels of dopamine and serotonin, known respectively as the pleasure chemical and the calming chemical. This is said to be part of the powerful addictive nature of nicotine, along with mood swings that come from withdrawal, when a person tries to quit smoking.

Lack of sleep – studies have shown that otherwise healthy people deprived of sleep had increased brain activity after viewing upsetting visual images than well-rested people. This was a reaction similar to that of depressed people. Poor sleep habits, therefore, could increase the risk of depression.

Thyroid disorder – hypothyroidism, a low-functioning or sluggish thyroid can lead to depression, since the butterfly-shaped gland in the neck is responsible for – among other things – regulating serotonin levels in the body. This condition can be treated with medication.

Unhappy relationships with siblings – according to a 2007 study in the American Journal of Psychiatry, men who did not get along well with brothers and/or sisters before age twenty were more likely to become depressed later in life than those with healthy sibling relationships.

Prescription medications – some anxiety and insomnia drugs, high blood pressure and cholesterol remedies, and others include depression as a possible side effect. Be aware of this possibility and always consult with your doctor.

Meanwhile, my new AA friends, Dave, Sandy, Ty, and others absolutely saved my life when they rescued me from that psycho woman. Even after I got away, though, and even after I met other women, I still tried to go back for more punishment.

One weekend after I had moved into the little mobile home, I had my baby daughter and her crazy mother convinced me to also watch her three other kids while she went to work. As soon as her shift at the restaurant ended, she said, she would come over and pick them up. Sure, I agreed, no problem, and I packed everybody up in my car and went to spend the evening at home, watching TV.

By around midnight, with no word from her, I left the older girl in charge – she was probably twelve or thirteen by now – and drove over to the rental house near the lake where I used to live with the Evil One. The porch light was on, and there were two cars in the driveway, one of which was hers.

I went up and knocked on the door, heard a bunch of running around inside. Knocked some more; heard more running around, footsteps thump-thumping off the raised wooden floor. Finally, the door opened and there she was, asking me what I wanted.

"Yes, a guy is here," she said, "sleeping on the couch."

This woman had conned me into babysitting her kids so she could bring another man home to spend the night. It took me a while, but I finally realized that all I was ever really good for in the first place was two things: an extra paycheck and free babysitting.

Like I said, she saw my dumb ass coming a mile away. I was one in a long line of suckers. My daughter told me a few years ago that one time she and her (half) sister were talking about it, and by the time they finished counting the number of men in and out of the house during their lifetimes, they reached a total of thirty-seven.

Amazing. Sad but true.

The worst part, though? I still wanted to get back together with this person.

I remember one afternoon talking to a friend named Jesse about it. By then, I was seeing a very nice girl who treated me like a king, I told him, and yet I still wanted the crazy one who made my life absolutely miserable.

Jesse looked at me like the idiot that I was:

"Let me get this straight," he said, with sort of a smirk on his face. "You've got one woman who treats you like a king, and one who treats you like shit. Where is the decision, man?"

Eventually, I got over my pitiful obsession, although I had to put up with this woman's shenanigans for another sixteen years – and voluntarily pay her child support (there was no court order) – until my daughter turned eighteen. That was five years ago, and I've neither seen nor spoken to her since. It has been wonderful.

One Saturday in May, after I screwed up the relationship with the woman who treated me like a king, I was covering local elections at city hall, standing around shooting the breeze with other media types, waiting for voting returns to come in, and I asked a female reporter I knew from one of the local radio stations if she had any single friends. She said that she did not, but she might know someone who did. She made a phone call, talked to one of her female friends, and the next I knew, I had a number.

It may have been later that night or the next night, I called that number and got a voice mail message. Really nice voice. So I left a message – she knew from her friend who provided the number that I would be calling – and she called me back, and we agreed to go out that next Friday night.

We met outside a convenience store, and the blind date went really well. We were basically together from then on, either talking on the phone or going out. Both of us were damaged goods, and so the road was often rocky, but we stuck it out, plowed through some hard times, and came out on the other side, happier than ever and still together twenty years later.

About three or four years after we started seeing each other, I received the worse news of my life.

My mother had brain cancer.

It was my sister who told me in a phone call that doctors had found "a mass" in my mother's brain. She was crying and saying, "We can't lose our mama."

My head was spinning. I called my mother and she sounded like her usual cheerful and happy self. Yes, she had a tumor, she said, but it was small – the size of a pea, she said – and they were going to operate, remove it, and everything was going to be fine.

It turned out that was a bunch of bullshit, since what she actually had was a good-sized glioblastoma, a nasty type of malignancy with an extremely dismal survival rate. But she said everything was going to be fine, and that was good enough for me.

What she was doing, of course, was trying to spare her kids the awful news that their mother was dying. I'm not sure how I would have reacted if she had told me the truth, but I always believed my mama, and this was a lot easier to swallow.

There were signs pretty quickly that I should have picked up on, like her letting me know she was getting such things as her will and other paperwork in order, having me sign a medical power of attorney agreement that authorized me to make healthcare decisions on her behalf, if necessary, and pushing and pushing for all of us to go on a family camping trip to Galveston Island State Park.

One of her grandmothers had lived in Galveston at one time, she had lived there for a few years as a young girl while her father inspected incoming ships at the port, and living an hour's drive away in Houston most of her life, it was one of mama's favorite places in the world. Her unusual and persistent eagerness to get all us kids together and spend a weekend down there for the first time ever should have raised my suspicions a little, but I did not want to believe my mother was gravely ill, and so I didn't.

We had the family camp-out, and she underwent brain surgery, which was horrendous. The whole timeline is kind of fuzzy now, but I remember going to her house at Christmas, which was always great fun, and seeing her kind of shuffle into the living room, smiling, with one side of her head completely shaved, revealing a huge, ugly, red, horseshoe-shaped incision closed with lots and lots of staples.

She was on some heavy medication, but in good spirits, or at least putting on a brave face.

Although she improved some at first – they had not been able to remove all the tumor – in the end, she started wasting away and I think the final round of chemotherapy is what finally killed her.

The last image I have of my mother is her lying in a hospital bed at her house in tiny Iola, Texas, eyes closed, mostly unresponsive, although her face crinkled up and she started crying when I leaned over and told her I loved her. The thing about that mental picture that strikes me the most is her right hand, steadfastly clutching one of the rails on that hospital bed.

She was basically in a coma, I guess, but holding on to life with everything she had.

A week later, my father called me at work and did not come right out and say it, but I could tell that he was trying to tell me something, and I finally figured out what it had to be. The room spun a little bit, as I stood and looked around, trying to figure out what to do next. My boss knew what was going on, so I called and told him I was taking off.

Then I called my sister, who lived in the same little town as our mother, about a hundred-fifty miles from me, and told her I would be on my way down there right away.

"Why?" she said, her voice cold as ice. "It's too late now. You're such an asshole, John. What makes you think I need you?"

"Because we're family," I said. "Please don't do this."

"Don't bother," she answered, and hung up.

If unhappy relationships with siblings is part of the recipe for developing depression, this family could have been a test case.

My sister and I hated each other the whole time we were growing up. Not just sibling rivalry. This was intense dislike. I don't know where that comes from, exactly. She told me one time after we were grown that it was hard growing up as my sister, since I was always popular and successful, an overachiever at everything. It was one of those stereotypical situations you hear about – "Oh, you're John's sister!"

She was daddy's little girl to an extreme, especially after she nearly died from a case of encephalitis when she was two years old, and I was my mother's favorite. Our little brother was left somewhere out in left field. That's probably why he stayed in so much trouble. Any kind of attention – even negative and often painful attention – was better than nothing, I suppose.

There was never any love lost between any of us. Here's a little example of how we all got along:

One day playing in the next-door neighbor's backyard, I kicked my sister in the head – I don't remember why; she was on the ground and I kicked her – and got in a lot of trouble.

As an attempted payback for telling on me, I squirted a healthy shot of liquid dish soap into a pitcher of orange juice I found sitting on the kitchen counter, next to the sink. For some reason, I knew or suspected my sister was about to drink some, and sure enough, she did.

Naturally, she howled and spit and sputtered. For some reason, my little brother was the primary suspect, and although he vigorously denied any wrongdoing, I let him take the heat, and the beating that went with it.

Our home was a war zone throughout my teenage years, and I hauled ass as soon as I graduated. Any plans I had for the future were long gone, and my only ambition at that point was getting loaded every day.

I was highly successful at that, and my sister and brother followed suit.

The three of us traveled in familiar circles, had a few mutual friends, and so spent time together occasionally, mostly revolving around the consumption of mind-altering substances.

Whatever relationship we might have had, however, collapsed when our mother died.

When I drove down for the memorial service, I found out that my sister, who was executrix of her estate, had ordered our mother immediately cremated. My mother wanted to be cremated, but it would have been nice to hold off on that at least long enough for me and my brother to be able to see her one last time and say good-bye.

My dear sister purposely stole that chance from me. For me, mama was here one day and poof! gone the next. Just disappeared. For me, it's like she is away somewhere on vacation, but she never comes back.

It was my fault for not talking to her about final arrangements while she was alive, but I was in complete denial most of the time she was sick. And I never dreamed my sister would do such a thing. I still wish there were a place I could go and visit her some times. Sit next to a grave and feel somewhat close to her, maybe have a little chat.

I have no idea what happened to the urn of ashes, which was given to my brother at the memorial service, and wound up in my sister's hands later that day.

That is not what ultimately destroyed our relationship forever, though. As I said, dear sister was executrix of the estate, which was not a staggering amount of wealth, by any means, but consisted of two houses, more than one hundred acres of land and other investments. I know for a fact that my mother went to a lot of trouble to make sure everything was divided between the three kids, and I had no reason to think her wishes would not be carried out.

Unfortunately, they were not.

When all was said and done, I wound up with a grand total of $7,500. The rest − at least a couple of hundred thousand dollars in cash and real estate, I would imagine − was stolen by my sister. After I finally figured out what was going on, I met with attorneys two different times to see what I could do, but no luck.

Too much time had passed, I was told, and pursuing the case would be expensive and probably unsuccessful in the end. Apparently, the will had been amended shortly before my mother's death, even though she was in no condition herself to do so.

Not only that, my sister and brother somehow wound up with mineral rights to all the property formerly owned by our mother, and oil was discovered a few years ago. Now, they both get fat checks in the mail every month, and I, of course, get nothing.

In our last "conversation," which was actually via Facebook messaging, my lovely sister told me that mama wanted me cut out of the will: "Fuck you, John! She didn't want you to have any of her money. You're the reason she's dead!"

Needless to say, there has been no contact since, with either my sister or brother.

I can be such a naïve fool sometimes. I really can.

So the day of the memorial service came. It was at a little country church, down a narrow dirt road through the woods from mama's house. I walked in through a door that opened into the kitchen, which was connected to the main chapel.

I walked through the kitchen, took a few steps inside the chapel, and saw a small table covered with a white cloth and filled with framed family photographs. That is when the reality started to sink in, and I began to feel a little overwhelmed. For the first time, it hit me that my mother was really gone – permanently. She was not there. The only thing left of her was a bunch of pictures on a little table.

I saw my nephew, Matt, sitting far across the room, bent over and sobbing, with somebody next to him, their arm around his shoulders.

Emotions started to rise. The back of my throat hurt, and I had to concentrate to be able to choke everything back down. I thought if I started to cry, I would never be able to stop.

Along with a nice eulogy by the local minister – whose words comforted me quite a bit when he mentioned that my mother had lived a good life, which was something I hadn't really thought about at that point – the three of us kids were given a chance to speak.

I think my brother went first, and all I remember about his talk was him shouting the word, "Acceptance," as he stood up to the podium, then a bunch of crazy bullshit. My sister told some ridiculous self-serving story about mama calling one of her grandsons "my little cookie man," because he brought her a chocolate chip cookie one time, or some such crap.

When it was my turn, I walked up and pulled a piece of paper out of my pocket. Almost as soon as I found out about the "mass" in her brain, I shut myself up in what I then called my music room and wrote an essay called "Mama Died Today." It was my way of dealing with things.

I decided I would read that at her service.

I unfolded the sheet of paper and laid it on the podium, looked out at the audience for the first time, and said something inane, like "Wow, there's a lot of people here."

Then I looked down at the essay, which began with her name, "Billie Jo Jones."

I could not speak. I could not say her name. I was taking deep breaths and trying to calm myself, but the words would not come. I knew if I said anything, the floodgates would be unleashed and I would become a crying puddle on the floor, in front of God and everybody.

It took what seemed like five minutes, at least, before I could squeeze out the words, "Billie Jo Jones was born in San Pedro, California …"

I talked about her going to Milby High School in Houston, and swimming on the school swim team; about her taking us kids to the movies, making Christmas cookies, and teaching me how to cook, especially how to make those great cherry pies.

After the service, and the little reception or whatever, where everybody sits around and eats and tells stories, the family went back to mama's house for a while, and then it was all over.

Chapter Ten

So, are you really depressed?

Most people feel sad sometimes, discouraged, bummed out – but for some of us, this type of mood does not go away. One way to tell if you might have a problem is to ask yourself whether whatever it is you are feeling is affecting your daily life in a negative way.

Ask yourself:

Do you have trouble falling asleep at night?

Are you often extra tired, feeling run-down?

Have you gained or lost weight without explanation?

Has your sex drive decreased?

Does depression run in your family?

Do you try and avoid people?

Do you hate getting out of bed in the morning?

Do you think feeling unhappy is normal, and wonder how people who appear to be happy do it?

Do you ever ask yourself what is the point of going on?

If you answered yes to some or all of those questions, there is a chance you may have a problem. The good news, though, is that the problem is entirely fixable.

Depression can be overcome.

One common way people try to feel better is with medication. Sometimes there are unpleasant side effects, and many times, the medications simply do not work.

I have tried four or five of the most commonly prescribed anti-depressants, and none of them ever did a thing to help. One of them – I don't remember which – seemed to have some positive effect, but it also completely killed my sex drive and function, so that was out. Being unable to have sex is *really* depressing.

A lot of people, however, apparently do well on various medications, so it is always a good idea to consult a physician. You can start with your regular family doctor. Do your research before you go, and be aware that most likely, the doc is going to whip out the prescription pad and send you to the drug store, prescribing this or that, in hopes you feel better and there you go. Nothing inherently wrong with that approach. That's just what they do.

You also might be referred to a psychiatrist, who has more knowledge about psychotropic drugs, but be aware that some of those are extremely powerful brain altering substances and should not be taken lightly.

Although medication has never worked for me, serious depression sometimes can apparently be caused by a chemical imbalance in the brain, and medication is the only answer. If that is the solution that works best for you, then by all means, do it.

By all means, please do it.

Another possible treatment option is counseling. If you are anything like me – an emotional cripple, of sorts – having someone to help you sort out your feelings and emotions, understand why you are feeling the way you are, can go a long way toward lightening your load and brightening your outlook.

Talk to a close friend or relative, see what they think. Simply getting things off your chest may be just the ticket to leave you feeling happier and more hopeful.

A lot of times, it is that one deep, dark secret – maybe more than one – that can wreak havoc in our lives. Remember, other people go through shit in this life, too. You are not the only one. You are never alone.

When I was first going through the recovery steps of AA, one of the procedures is to meet with someone and tell them your deepest, darkest, most shameful secrets. Remember, things like alcohol and drug abuse are only a symptom of deeper, darker underlying problems.

Getting those things out of hiding, into the open air, eliminating that horrible guilt, regret and shame, can go a long way toward progressing in your recovery.

For me, I had one deep, dark, dirty secret in particular that I could not imagine actually telling another human being, no matter who they were. My sponsor – the guy with the seven DWIs – finally gave up after I kept resisting this crucial step, and asked his sponsor to take over.

This guy, named Richard, was tall and outgoing, confident, good-looking and charismatic. The kind of guy to whom people have a hard time saying no.

He grabbed me after a meeting one night and said, "Come over to my house Saturday, and we'll do your fifth step. Here's the address. See you at ten o'clock."

Gulp.

I met with him, and we both knew I didn't want to do it.

Richard looked at me and said, "C'mon, look, when I was a kid, I used to fuck watermelons. Whatever you did is no big deal."

So I took a deep breath and told him my secret.

What a relief.

One thing you need to do for sure is get things off your chest. You and your problems are not unique, and you're not alone.

With today's technology, you can even go talk to someone virtually, and hide safely behind your laptop. Look for online support groups, forums, chat rooms. You can preserve your anonymity and still find a sympathetic ear.

Another thing you can do is to simply become more active. Go for a walk – a long one. Even if you don't feel like it. The human body is designed to move, and it loves to walk. There is a four-mile route down and around some country roads where I live, and it takes right at an hour to complete the circuit from my driveway and back, and it feels really good, physically and mentally.

Now, back to the story:

Within about a year after mama died, I started getting really restless. My world had changed in a big way.

I didn't know it at the time, but I was changing, too.

It didn't happen overnight, but I was no longer enjoying the job I had loved for the past twelve or thirteen years, which should probably have been seen as a sign, but I had no idea about depression then. Like I said, I really didn't even believe in depression as any sort of medical condition.

Remember, the way I was raised was to just get over it. Feel bad? Well, hell, that's easy. Don't feel that way.

Next!

I thought it was my job that was making me unhappy, so I started thinking about what I could do besides newspaper reporting. I just didn't have any enthusiasm anymore for going out and chasing down stories.

Where I lived – and still live – is an area where the economy is dominated by Fort Hood, the largest military installation in the country. Around here, people pretty much work in some kind of military-related job, for local government agencies, school districts and the service industry.

Some of my former colleagues had become school teachers, and that didn't sound like a bad idea, especially considering all the news at the time about teacher shortages.

I really couldn't see myself doing something like that, though, so I kept going to work, hating it, and not doing a whole helluva lot, to tell you the truth. I'd put out a few stories a week – at one time, I was known to put out several stories a day – but it's a wonder I never caught any flak from the main office.

And I kept thinking about the teaching thing. I wanted a change so badly, and I told myself that teaching is a noble profession, and would be a good legacy to leave. Spending a couple decades of one's life as a teacher would not be a bad thing at all.

I could not imagine, however, standing in front of a classroom, talking all day. I hate to talk. I am a writer. I write. Not talk.

Finally, I started going to people I trusted and asking what they thought about the whole thing. All the responses were positive, and so I started looking into what it would take to get my state teaching license.

Then, one day I called a woman named Dr. Ann Farris, who at the time was deputy superintendent for a local school district. I made an appointment to see her, and when I got there, she took me to a meeting room, where we sat next to each other at one end of a long conference table.

I told her what I was up to, and she said, "Well, I think you would make a great teacher."

"What makes you say that?" I asked.

"Because you're a good man," she said, looking me in the eye.

The way she said it, and the way she looked at me, touched my heart and put a lump in my throat. I told myself, "Don't you dare cry in front of this woman."

I'm not sure exactly what else was said, but I thanked her and left, convinced that if this woman thought I could do it, then maybe I could.

I applied at a local branch of Tarleton State University for an alternative teaching certification program that caters to people who already have a college degree, but need to meet a few additional requirements to be able to take the state certification exam.

About six months later, I quit my job, wrapped up the final courses over the summer, and the next thing you know, I was a junior high school reading teacher.

I was hired the day before school started, which was a little nerve-wracking, since I had always heard there was a tremendous teacher shortage in Texas, and I wasn't getting any offers all through the summer. But then I got my shot, and I remember being in my new classroom, arranging desks and such, when the principal who hired me walked in. I asked him what I was supposed to do the first day, thinking he would hand me some sort of manual full of the stuff I was supposed to teach.

I will never forget what he said:

"Don't worry about it. It'll come to you."

What? Don't worry about it? It'll come to me? You've got to be kidding! These desks are going to filled with teenagers tomorrow, man, and I don't have a fucking clue what to do with them.

Luckily, I was surrounded by some wonderful veteran teachers who started handing me things to help me get started.

"Here, do this."

"Take these."

"You can use those."

Things went okay that first year, but what I found out was that a career change was not the solution for what was going on inside me. A new job was not the cure for what ailed, and it was not getting any better.

I was terribly unhappy, wondering if I'd made a bad decision with my new career, wondering about my sometimes rocky marriage about four years before, and just generally a mess.

So, for the first time in my life, I sought counseling.

Chapter Eleven

The last time I went for some counseling, not too long ago, the very nice young lady – who was enjoyable enough to talk to, but had no idea what to do with me – gave me during our second and final session a one-page list of "thinking errors" that can produce a negative mindset, and generally shitty outlook on life.

Here is that list:

All or nothing thinking (also called black-and-white, polarized or dichotomous thinking): when you view a situation in only two categories, instead of on a continuum.

Anticipating negative outcomes: Expecting that something negative has happened or is going to happen. Two types of thinking errors fall into this particular category:

• **Fortune telling**: Predicting that something negative is going to happen in the future, as if you are gazing into a crystal ball.

• **Catastrophizing**: Telling yourself that the very worst is happening or is going to happen, without considering other possibilities that may be more likely and/or less negative.

Disqualifying or discounting the positive: Unreasonably telling yourself that positive experiences, deeds or qualities do not count.

Emotional reasoning: Thinking something must be true because you "feel" (actually, believe) it so strongly, ignoring or discounting evidence to the contrary.

Labeling: Putting a fixed, global label on yourself or others without considering that the evidence might more reasonably lead to a less disastrous conclusion.

Mental filter (also called selective abstraction): Paying undue attention to one negative detail instead of seeing the whole picture.

Mind reading: Believing you know what others are thinking, failing to consider other, more likely, possibilities, and making no effort to check it out.

Overgeneralization: Making a sweeping negative conclusion that goes far beyond the current situation.

"Should" and "must" statements (also called imperatives): Having a precise, fixed idea of how you or others should behave and overestimating how bad it is that these expectations are not met.

Maladaptive thoughts: Problematic thoughts that do not contain logical thinking errors. These thoughts may be true. However, dwelling on them makes you feel more anxious and may interfere with your performance.

A lot of those apply to me, no question about it.

I definitely tend to look at things as black and white, with little or no gray area. I find it difficult to "agree to disagree." Normal-minded, well-adjusted people can easily accomplish this, but I tend to blow things out of proportion; make too big a deal out of it; take things personally.

In my mind, if you disagree with me, then you are criticizing me fundamentally as a person. And if I cannot persuade you to come over to my side, so to speak, then there is a rift between us that may be insurmountable.

Political debates, for example. I have friends with whom I am completely at odds when it comes to certain issues. We don't agree at all on some things, and I tend to wonder how we can be friends and still have these tremendous differences in thought and belief. They, on the other hand, don't take it to heart; don't take my disagreeing with them as a personal attack. It is just a discussion item, an issue.

Anticipating negative outcomes. Well, I think we've already discovered I have quite the capacity for negativity. I came by it naturally, and it is so deeply ingrained in my thinking processes that it is one of my biggest challenges.

Like my mother told me that night at the hospital, "Don't borrow trouble, son."

Such a simple idea, and yet so complex.

Discounting the positive: all the things I have accomplished in my life, and nothing is ever good enough. I know in my heart of hearts that if I were to discover the cure for cancer, become world-famous, loved by all, and filthy rich, I would not be satisfied. I don't know exactly why that is, but I'm pretty confident it is true.

Emotional reasoning: all my life, I have sort of confused reality with fantasy. I imagined things were the way I wanted them to be, and failed to see things the way they actually were. Remember my photographer friend asking me when I was going to get rid of my white horse, when I was driving myself completely insane thinking I was going to ride in to that poor woman's life and save her from herself?

Puh-leeze.

Another unrealistic and twisted thing I have always done is to base my opinion of myself on other people's opinion of me. If someone did not like me, in my mind, there must be something wrong with me.

The first time I heard something about myself that I could identify with, that made sense to me, was in an AA meeting a long time ago, when someone referred to themselves as "an egomaniac with an inferiority complex."

Wow, I thought, that's me. An egomaniac with an inferiority complex. I think I am better than a lot of people – better-looking, more intelligent, more successful – and a piece of shit at the same time.

It takes a special individual to think they are both superior and inferior to someone all at once.

Labeling: good grief, how long does this list go on? I am a king of labelers; judgmental. That old saying about not judging a book by its cover? Hell, if I don't like the cover, I don't even bother to read the book.

I still do this a whole lot more than I should.

Another crazy thing I still do is to quickly put people on my shit list and keep them there. You know that old song, "One, two, three strikes you're out, at the old ballgame?" Well, with me making the rules, you're quite likely to be out after only one strike.

I did not speak to a co-worker for two years after she said something critical about me that I did not like. Never mind the fact that it was true. As I write this very sentence, another one of my co-workers has been on my shit list for three weeks, and most likely does not have a clue why. She knows I am not speaking to her, but I'm sure she has no idea the reason.

Mental filter: focusing on the negative instead of anything positive about a given situation. Check.

Mind reading: if I could read minds as well as I think I can, I would definitely be rich and famous. Check. Overgeneralization, check. Should and must statements, check. Maladaptive thoughts, check.

Sheesh. Not only do some of the things on the thinking errors list apply to me, they all do. Can one seemingly normal person really be so screwed up?

But back to the first time I sought counseling.

I made an appointment with the mental health department at a mega-hospital in my area, and the first time I went there, I filled out some paperwork, and in short order they took me into a room where I did some computerized evaluations and other stuff, and the verdict came back that I suffered from mild depression and anxiety.

When I saw my therapist for the first time, he was fascinated by my IQ level, which was apparently a part of the evaluation and something I won't reveal here. Let's just say I'm at the upper levels on the intelligence scale, and this guy was talking about how rare and interesting it was for him to have someone like that come in.

So, having a high IQ means a person is less susceptible to developing depression?

It figures that I would be one of the exceptions.

I went for several sessions with this guy and enjoyed it, but then summer came and school let out, and I quit going, as he predicted I eventually would.

Chapter 12

So, what exactly is the link between one's intelligence level and depression? Is there a link?

A good friend named Jim once told me: "Human beings are the only animals in the world that sit around scratching their asses saying, 'Why am I here?'"

It's true. All other animals go about their business every day, doing what they do, living their lives, without all the crazy contemplation and self-examination about the meaning of life, creation of the universe, what happens after they die, all that stuff. They just eat and sleep and live.

Another of my friends, who I know does not consider himself a particularly wise man, said this incredibly wise thing one time when I told him I was struggling with figuring out who I am, and what I am all about.

"You know yourself better than you think," he said. "Here's what you need to do: Live more and think less."

Live more and think less.

Five incredibly powerful words.

Just think about it.

According to some studies, there is a positive relationship between low intelligence levels and depression. Not high intelligence, but low. In other words, it may be true that people with low IQ are less happy than people with high IQ.

There are, however, researchers who claim the opposite is true.

Of course there are.

I, not a professional researcher, can definitively say that higher levels of intelligence are not a protection from depression. Just look at me for proof, and I would guess that my sister and brother also have fairly high IQs, and, well, I don't think I need to say anything else about that.

One study I found suggested that having a high IQ leads people to "re-create" their actual world with a world that better suits their likes and dislikes. Sounds similar to what I was talking about with my tendency to imagine things being a certain way, while ignoring the painfully obvious reality right in front of me, thereby producing a more comfortable world that I could understand and deal with better.

Sounds a little crazy, actually, but we press on.

Another characteristic of at least some highly intelligent people is the tendency to be sensitive, and socially withdrawn.

Ahem.

I am both overly sensitive, and way too socially withdrawn.

Guilty on each count.

In my defense, research suggests there are reasons for both.

I love to be able to justify my objectionable behavior.

Apparently, that inner dialogue confusing fantasy with reality that some high IQ folks engage in distracts them from finding like-minds with whom they can relate on a similar intellectual and/or emotional level. This can produce a feeling of alienation from the world that leads to such things as depression.

That was probably the case for a long time with me, especially considering I was in a persistent state of semi-consciousness for more than a decade. Who better to hang out and spend time with than a bunch of other screwed-up people? And I hung out with some real doozies back in the day.

In recent years, though, I have allowed myself to open up enough to have a few close friends who actually love and care about me, inspire me, and make me want to be a better man.

I give a lot of credit for that to some really amazing people, including my brothers, Bobby and Joe, who are not true blood-brothers, but lifelong friends closer to me in many ways than so-called family.

Bobby and I grew up about a mile apart, a short walk and even shorter bicycle ride from his house to mine. We went to the same schools from kindergarten through twelfth grade, played sports together, our parents were friends. I met Joe in junior high, when we both tried out for seventh-grade basketball.

I lost touch with both these guys after high school, until a chance conversation via the Internet with a an old high school classmate led me to find out Bobby was head of his own company in Sugarland, Texas, so I looked up the phone number and called him.

Not long after that, I drove down there on a vacation day from work, found his offices – actually a large manufacturing complex – and walked inside what appeared to be the main building. A very nice receptionist showed me to Bobby's office, and voila, there he was.

My childhood friend, walking out from behind his desk with a big smile and outstretched hand, looked basically the same, except he was dressed like a businessman, and now he had short hair.

Other than that, even though it had been thirty years since we'd seen each other, it was like no time had passed.

Bobby showed me around his offices, the warehouse, and the massive manufacturing operation out back, and then we went to lunch at a Chinese restaurant before heading over to a local country club for an afternoon round of golf.

Shortly after I walked in earlier that morning, Bobby was on the phone to Joe, telling him I was standing there, and that he had to take off the rest of the day to play some golf. It took a little coaxing to get Joe to take the afternoon off from work, but when we got to the golf course, there he was, leaning against the trunk of his car, lacing up his golf shoes.

Joe and Bobby had remained close friends over the years, while I took off in another direction after high school, but we had a great time playing golf and vowed to do it again soon.

That meeting led to another and another, then the first of what has become semi-annual boys' weekends down in Galveston, where Bobby owns a magnificent beach house a couple hundred yards from the Gulf of Mexico. Birthday celebrations. Holiday dinners.

One spring morning the three of us were sitting in the kitchen/dining area of Bobby's beach house, drinking coffee and talking about old times, when the subject of our renewed friendship came up, and nobody could really explain the near-instant bond that had formed after so many years.

"I don't know," said Bobby, a master salesman and public speaker who is never, ever at a loss for words. "It just works."

For a while, I didn't really trust their friendship. I thought maybe they were just being nice, not wanting to hurt my feelings. Why would these great guys want to have anything to do with me?

Bobby is set-for-life wealthy, while Joe is easily one of the nicest people to ever walk the planet. Why bother with a screwed-up person like me?

Finally, I figured it out.

They enjoy spending time with me for the same reason(s) I enjoy spending time with them. Simply put, we have a good time together; enjoy each other's company. Nothing overly dramatic or complicated about it, and nothing that needs to be dissected by a paranoid, insecure, neurotic mind like mine.

For me, they make me feel good, inside and out. They make me want to be a better person, and I am, in some ways. It is not macho to say, but I love them and they love me.

Pretty simple.

As far as the overly-sensitive part, here's a story that represents a fine example. This is a blog I wrote as a contributor to Liyahamore Publishing, an outfit I discovered by chance and started writing for twice a week.

"Several years ago, a woman reported to her boss what she believed to be misbehavior on the part of one of her co-workers, and that co-worker was subsequently reprimanded.

Nothing major, but an official slap on the wrist and documentation in the employee file.

That co-worker was me, and I did not speak to that woman for two years after that.

It wasn't so much that she found fault with the way I handled a certain situation – everyone is entitled to their opinion – but how dare she go behind my back with bad intent. After leaving the boss' office that morning, I figured out a handful of suspects who could have been involved, and I asked them one by one if they had gone to the big office to complain about me.

Everyone denied it, until I got to the last person on the list. To her credit, she looked me straight in the eye and admitted it. She was still trying to explain when I turned around and walked out of the room, never to return, never intending to speak to her again.

That is a good example of how I handle conflict.

Not a good example of how to handle conflict, mind you, but an example of how I tend to do it.

There's an old baseball song called "Take Me Out to the Ballgame," and one line in the song says, 'For it's one, two, three strikes, you're out …"

In baseball, you get three chances to get it right.

With me a lot of times, it's one strike and you're out.

Not exactly the right way to manage a problem.

Ephesians 4:31-32 says, "Let all bitterness and wrath and anger and clamor and slander be put away from you, along with all malice. Be kind to one another, tender-hearted, forgiving one another, as God in Christ forgave you."

One of the reasons for forgiveness, of course, is that holding on to bitterness and resentment takes work. It can be stressful, and perpetual stress is not good for body and soul.

Carrying that grudge around hurts the grudge-holder the most. The target of those hard feelings has most likely moved on, happily living their life, while you are still back there fuming and stewing and holding on to the past.

Here's an idea.

Let it go.

Just let it go.

If that's too tough, I have heard but never been able to make myself try another oft-recommended solution – pray for the person who wronged you.

Matthew 5:44 says, "But I tell you, love your enemies and pray for those who persecute you."

I don't know about you, but I find it a real challenge to pray for someone who shoved a knife in my back – or worse – and is now merrily going about their business. Pray for them to get hit by a truck maybe, but that is not what the scripture intends.

Someone told me long ago that if I could not think of anything positive to pray for, I could ask God that my enemy "get everything they deserve." I think God could see through that one.

Instead, we are to ask for God's grace and blessings on the person we would really enjoy throttling. Along with avoiding possible criminal charges, this approach also brings God's loving grace to us. I have always heard that praying daily for two consecutive weeks for someone with whom you are having a conflict will reduce or even remove those resentments that are hurting you a lot more than they are hurting them.

And as a side benefit, you'll be praying every day, which is never a bad idea.

Let me say here that I am not a regular practitioner of prayer, or even meditation. I don't go to church and I don't much care for organized religion.

I do, however, enjoy writing for this Bible-based website because there are good things to be learned from the scriptures; good things to remember while trying to become a better person.

Hell, it sure can't hurt anything.

Chapter 13

A lot of my story so far, it seems, has been about alcohol abuse.

Does one thing lead to another?

Does depression lead to alcohol abuse, or does alcohol abuse lead to depression?

Yes.

Huh?

Well, which came first, the chicken or the egg?

According to everydayhealth.com, common signs of depression in people abusing alcohol include such things as sadness and hopelessness, changes in sleep habits or appetite, loss of interests in once pleasurable activities, guilt, feelings of worthlessness, and suicidal thoughts.

Sounds about the same as symptoms for alcohol-free depression.

One of the problems, when you try and treat depression with alcohol, is that both problems can get worse.

An American Foundation for Suicide Prevention report indicates the combination of alcohol and depression leads to more than seventy-five percent of all suicides. With someone who is experiencing untreated depression, the influence of alcohol – which is a nervous system depressant – can impair the person's ability to think clearly and cause them to impulsively take drastic and irreversible action to end the pain they are suffering.

Studies have shown that nearly a third of people with severe depression also have a drinking problem. Many times, it is the depression that comes first. In children, for example, depression sufferers are more likely to develop alcohol problems, and teenagers with depression are twice as likely to abuse alcohol as those who have not suffered. Women with a history of depression, too, are at greater risk than men for heavy drinking.

Needless to say, alcohol makes depression worse. Heavy consumption can also make antidepressant medications less effective.

It is said that if you think you may have a drinking problem, you probably do. Same thing with depression. If you think you may be depressed, you probably are. In either case, the first step is to see physician. Both conditions are treatable, and not signs of weakness or some sort of character flaw.

Having the courage to recognize and admit a problem – or the possibility of a problem – and to seek help, is an act of not only courage, but wisdom and strength.

Several years ago, I was feeling shitty for a while and could not seem to shake it off, so I decided to try a little counseling again.

When I headed toward the door of the counseling offices, I walked by a woman standing outside, smoking a cigarette. She turned out to be my counselor. Actually, she was a licensed social worker, and I think I went back once, maybe twice, after that initial session, but it just wasn't working out. She seemed to be just checking the blocks, watching the clock, doing her job, and I didn't see any future in continuing.

Last year, I went for counseling again, and the young lady was nice enough, and seemed sincere in her desire to help people, but we both agreed during my second session that we really didn't have much to talk about. She is the one who gave me that list of thinking errors, which is really good and informative, in my opinion.

Over the years, I have also tried a handful of different medications prescribed by my general practitioner, including Zoloft, Effexor, Prozac, and either Paxil or Lexapro. None did anything to help.

About two years ago, I went to the doctor hoping to try something different, and he said that in light of so many previous unsuccessful attempts to find the right antidepressant, he was recommending an appointment with a psychiatrist, who would have more knowledge about medications and be better able to find the right drug.

I was all set with an appointment for a shrink, but then one day at work, a colleague asked me how I was doing, and instead of the usual, "Pretty good," or whatever, I told her the truth – that I wasn't doing so good.

She told me I needed to go talk to a mutual friend, with whom we worked.

I said okay and promptly forgot all about it, until he walked up to me a couple of days later and started asking me some questions. Then he told me he knew exactly why antidepressants had never worked for me.

He had been in the same boat for a long time, until he discovered testosterone replacement therapy. After he started taking weekly testosterone injections, he felt like a new man. I asked for the name of his doctor, and called that same day to make an appointment.

Testosterone levels naturally decrease as a man ages, some more severely than others. Among an array of related symptoms is depression, and my friend said the supplementation turned his life around.

It turned out, according to blood tests, that I did have significantly reduced levels of testosterone, and after the first injection in the doctor's office, I noticed a fairly dramatic improvement in my mood. I still inject myself once a week, although sometimes I run out because of simple laziness and because the stuff is somewhat expensive. When I go two or three weeks, I begin to experience noticeable fatigue, drop in energy levels and decline in mood. Basically, I start to feel like shit.

So, the testosterone definitely helps, but it hasn't been a magic bullet, either.

Right now, as I'm sitting in my office at home writing these very words, I can tell you that just last week, it dawned on me that I have been depressed for some time now, and doing way too much self-medicating.

I can tell you for sure that the self-medicating does not work. It does not work at all. Sure, you can go away for a while and maybe forget about your problems, but it is only a temporary solution that leaves you feeling worse than you felt before, physically and mentally.

Wait a second, you might be saying right about now, I thought you quit drinking back when you moved to Temple to go to work for that newspaper?

Yes, indeed, you are absolutely right.

I quit drinking for 22 years, and it saved my life. Most definitely.

Then, I went on a trip to Spain.

Chapter 14

Medical experts mostly agree that while people suffering from moderate to severe depression can experience good results using antidepressant medication, those with mild depression – like myself – may not respond as well.

According to an article published in health.com, for those folks who find that medication does not improve their situation, there are a number of non-drug remedies that may help. Such things as exercise, light therapy, journaling, acupuncture, support groups, and meditation have been shown to relieve depression.

One of the reasons I have fallen back into some bad habits, I believe, is simply a lack of physical activity.

I am a physical person. I enjoy being active, getting outdoors, playing sports, walking, hiking, working out at the gym, even mowing the grass. Unfortunately, about the only physical activity I have engaged in over the past several years is playing golf once a week. And, really, let's face it, playing golf is not that strenuous when you ride around the course in a golf cart.

There was a time when I was in great shape – lean, muscular, going to the gym every morning before work.

"Looking good, Billy Ray."

"Feeling good, Lewis."

Lines from the end of the excellent 1983 movie, Trading Places, starring Eddie Murphy and Dan Aykroyd. That was me, looking good and feeling good.

Now, I'm overweight, out of shape, and spend most of my spare time sitting in front of my laptop – which is a good thing, because I love to write – or laying on the couch, watching TV, which is not such a good thing.

I know I need to do something about my physical condition, and I know it would improve my mental state, but getting back into the groove is not an easy thing when you've been stuck in a deep rut for a long time.

There is no magic bullet, when it comes to exercise and health, and there is nothing easy about it. It takes effort, and it takes commitment.

If it has been a while since you've done any meaningful exercise, the first thing I would say is to go get a check-up. Go to the doctor for a little poking and prodding, just to make sure everything is hunky dory, and then go home and lace up those sneakers.

Go for a walk.

That's it. Go for a walk.

See if you can make one mile. Wear a watch or some kind of timer, and it will take you right around fifteen minutes to cover a mile, maybe a little longer. You may be a little sore the next day, or the day after, but that's a good thing. Muscle soreness from exercise lets you know you're on the right track.

Depending on how that first outing felt, gradually increase your distance and your pace the next time you go out. Don't overdo it, or you risk injury that may put you back on the sidelines and starting again from square one. Remember, along with those muscles that need to get toned up, there are lots of ligaments and tendons and things that are also not used to the stress and strain.

One of the most important things about exercise is that it needs to be consistent. It has to become a habit. And I know from experience that exercise is a habit that is much easier to break, than it is to form. So try and get out there every day, and work your way up to an hour of brisk walking.

According to the American Heart Association, it won't be long before you start to notice a whole gamut of positive changes, including relief from depression and anxiety.

The list includes: more energy, stress relief, better sleep quality, improved self-image, weight loss, and increased muscle strength, which can lead to further physical activity and even more improvement.

When you feel better physically, you feel better mentally.

So ... that trip to Spain.

That was five years ago now, and I guess I was experiencing a sort of mid-life crisis. I felt like I had really screwed up my life, made so many bad decisions, missed out on so many opportunities, wasted so much time.

I had friends who were business owners, millionaires, world travelers, champion athletes. Sure, I was successful in my own right – married, father, husband, college degree, good job, homeowner, money in the bank – but it wasn't enough. I spent a lot of time wondering, "What if ..."

I wanted to do something big; something great.

One thing I had read stories about that always sounded really cool and romantic to me was backpacking and riding the trains around Europe. I never imagined actually doing it – I had never been overseas – but a friend convinced me I could, and should.

So I started researching backpacking trips around Europe and discovered the Camino de Santiago pilgrimage, a 500-mile trek across northern Spain. I read articles and testimonials about it, talked with the wife, and decided this was something I wanted and needed to do.

For about six months, I went on longer and longer training walks, and read everything I could find about the Camino, joined a chat forum dedicated to the pilgrimage and bombarded people with questions, and then one day in June, I was on a plane headed across the Atlantic.

When I got to Madrid and stepped outside the airport terminal building, looking unsuccessfully for a bus to take me to Pamplona, I immediately started to question my decision. By the time I reached my hotel a few hours later, where I would spend two nights before starting my walk, I was seriously freaking out.

The first night wasn't so bad, probably since I was really tired from traveling, but the second night, faced with the prospect of strapping on my backpack the next morning, leaving the comfort and safety of the hotel, and walking out into the countryside toward who-knows-what, I had a pretty serious anxiety attack.

I was literally talking out loud to myself, trying to calm down, as I lay in bed in my tiny room, tossing and turning, my heart racing, my breathing labored.

"It's okay, John," I said, over and over. "You're gonna be okay. It's all right. You're gonna be okay."

I finally fell asleep sometime in the early morning hours, woke up around nine o'clock and headed out, feeling a little but not much better.

Of course, everything turned out fine, and the whole experience proved life-changing, as it does for a lot of people. I wrote a best-selling book about it, "Camino: Laughter and Tears Along Spain's 500-mile Camino de Santiago," if you're interested. Copies are available on amazon.com.

You can also visit my website at: www.johnhenryiii.com.

Oh, yeah, drinking again.

During my research on the Camino, I read things about Spanish culture, including food and drink, and how wine is considered an integral part of eating. I wish I had saved it, because I don't remember exactly how it went, but there was an expression in one of the articles that went something like this: "A meal without wine is not a meal."

I thought about it a lot, even talked to some friends about it, and finally decided that if I was going to immerse myself in Spanish culture for a month, I might as well go all the way. So that's the story of how and why I started drinking alcohol again during my first trip to Spain.

Pretty simple.

Honestly, it was liberating to get that non-drinking monkey off my back, so to speak. Contrary to what some say and believe, there was no monster waiting inside me to spring forth and destroy me after a few sips of alcohol. It did not have that power. Nothing to be afraid of, after all.

I enjoyed a frosty mug or two of San Miguel beer after a long day of walking. The vino tinto (red wine) over there is excellent, and always served with dinner. About halfway through my trip, a new friend suggested an after-dinner glass of brandy, which I had never tried before, and that was wonderful.

Same thing when I got back home. Everything was fine. I had not become a roaring, out-of-control drunk, getting wasted all the time, ruining my life. As a matter of fact, it wasn't long after I got back that I first became a published author.

Wanting to start making a little extra money, I answered an ad for proofreaders and editors, and wound up proofing books for a small start-up publishing company called Archangel Ink. This led to them publishing a book I had written a few years before, *Finding God: An Exploration of Spiritual Diversity in America's Heartland*.

That led to my Camino book being published, and then I went on a tear of cranking out books that resulted in eight titles produced over the next year. And now, this one.

I work full-time as a junior high English teacher, write a weekly column for a local newspaper, contribute two blogs a week to a friend's website, and also write books.

Next on the list is the story of my adventures last summer driving historic Route 66, from Chicago to Santa Monica, California.

So starting drinking again did not ruin my life.

I am a different person than I was way back when. Older; a little wiser. I know now how much I have to lose if I go off the deep end again.

Please understand that I am not recommending what I did for anybody else. Alcohol abuse is a serious thing, and like I said, if you think you might have a problem, you probably do. If it is something that is interfering with your life, then it may indeed be a problem.

Don't be afraid to ask for help.

Go talk to your doctor. Call someone. Look on-line for information about excessive drinking.

Like I said, it's not a sign of weakness.

Everybody has problems.

Not everybody is brave enough to admit it.

Chapter 15

After that first trip to Spain, I went back again two years later, partly to visit my friend, Tom, whom I met at dinner after my first day of walking and spent a lot of time with over the next few weeks.

Tom was born and raised in Norway, went to college in London, and then worked all over the world as a mechanical engineer, before retiring on the northwest coast of Spain. Although there is something like a twenty-year difference in our ages, we are so much alike it is uncanny.

And to think about the unlikelihood of us ever meeting is a little mind-boggling. How we just so happened to wind up at the same place, at the same time on the Camino de Santiago, at a little albergue in a small village called Uterga – everything that had to happen for our paths to cross – makes you wonder about coincidences and fate, divine intervention and all that.

One of the things I learned, especially during my first trip to Spain, was about facing and overcoming fear.

Fear is a powerful thing, and it often holds us back from doing things we really want to do. Some things I've read say that at the end of life, dying people regret the things they did not do, much more than they regret anything they did.

What I learned about fear is that fear is a good thing. It means you are alive. It means you are challenging yourself. If you never experience fear, it probably means you never take risks, never step outside your comfort zone.

If that sounds familiar, maybe you should try it sometime. Step outside your comfort zone. Do something you've always wanted to do, but thought you couldn't or shouldn't, or planned to do later.

Go ahead. The time is now.

Once I got over that initial anxiety of being alone in a foreign country, with limited command of the language, thousands of miles away from home, I was transformed. I felt strong and free, happier than I had been in a long, long time.

Not depressed at all.

I had faced and conquered tremendous fear, lived out of a backpack and walked seven days a week for four weeks across the country, met and befriended people from all over the world, and made it back home all in one piece.

Unfortunately, although I brought a lot of the Camino and lessons learned back home with me, I didn't really make much effort to nurture those positive things and help them grow, and eventually I slipped back into a lot of my old stinkin' thinkin' habits.

One thing that works against me is the fact that I have a very obsessive mind, which is apparently quite common in people who have anxiety. I have a tendency to focus on the negative, wish things were not the way they are, and dwell on silly, little things that don't really matter. I also have very thin skin and take things like slights and criticisms way too personally.

There was a time when I asked several of my close friends, "When you think of John Clark, what do you see?"

That is a lot to ask of someone, and a difficult question to answer. That was when my old journalist friend, Sig, told me that I needed to live more and think less.

Live more; think less.

Unfortunately, I am one of those crazy humans who thinks a lot – especially when I'm trying to go to sleep at night.

According to psychology, thousands of years ago, people didn't spend much time sitting around contemplating life, reliving the past, and worrying about the future. Trying to simply survive day to day was plenty to keep their minds occupied.

Over time, we started having more and more inner conversations, plotting against our enemies and chiding ourselves for our weaknesses. These inner conversations – mostly full of anger, worry, self-criticism – have a powerful emotional component, and are particularly difficult and even painful for those who are depressed, since the brain interprets this dialogue as an attack and initiates a call for survival that tells us to "submit."

Somehow, this signal to submit includes powerful negative feelings that are interpreted as depression. And since you are "under attack" by yourself, the brain never knows when the onslaught is over, because these thoughts refuse to stop. This is what leads – particularly in people with a high IQ, who may have very elaborate internal conversations – to a lifetime of ongoing suffering from depression.

During the past two years, I've gotten pretty far down in the dumps more than a few times, and self-medicated a bit too much at times, as well. But I haven't let things get completely out of hand.

One of my major problems – probably *the* major problem – is feeling trapped in a job that I do not enjoy. Life can become a drudgery when you hate getting up in the morning to go to work. That is pretty much why my last attempt at counseling only lasted two sessions. There really wasn't much to talk about, other than the fact that my job was making me miserable.

So why don't I go out and get a new job, right?

Well, that's a trade-off.

Do I continue with a job that is mostly unsatisfying, unfulfilling, and not something I enjoy, or try and find something else that makes me happier, but in all likelihood, pays a lot less and affords me almost no vacation time, compared to teaching school.

Climbing back down the ladder of success.

That is what I mean about being stuck.

There are good parts to what I do for a living. The hours are good. Pay is not great, but decent. I get something like sixteen weeks' vacation a year. But me, of course, I tend to focus on the negative, and let the bad things overwhelm me. In reality, I have it pretty darned good.

And the truth is, there is no perfect job.

Well, maybe professional golfer. Unfortunately, I'm not anywhere near good enough and way too old to give that a go.

I have been successful in three different careers since I graduated high school, and I'm at the age now – late 50s – where it's a little late in the game to think about starting over yet again. So I try and focus instead on my writing, which makes me happy and fulfilled.

I have a lot to be thankful for, which is something I frequently forget to remember. I have a woman who loves and takes care of me. I have two daughters who are healthy and happy, making their own way in the world. I have two step-sons who think of me as a second father and called me "Pops." I have some incredible friends who inspire and even let me hang out with them once in a while. I have a roof over my head, food on the table, and the time and the wherewithal to travel pretty much wherever I want to go.

And don't let me forget the big one – I have my health.

One of my closest friends in the world recently underwent major surgery for prostate cancer. Everything is okay now, but I spent two days visiting him at MD Anderson Cancer Center in Houston, and it was an eye-opening experience, seeing so many sick, sick people walking up and down the corridors and riding elevators, attached to rolling IV racks, often with someone holding on to an arm to help keep them steady.

Waiting rooms full of people sitting somewhat patiently and quite expectantly – half a day sometimes – waiting for surgeries to be finished, and doctors to come report good news about how things turned out.

I came away from those two days with a profound sense of gratitude that until just this moment I was starting to let slip away. Compared to those folks, I have not a damn thing to complain about.

I have been through a lot of shit during my life, but everything that ever happened to me has led me to where I am right now, and, friends, I tell you what, it ain't a half-bad place.

Conclusion

"If I feel depressed, I will sing.
"If I feel sad, I will laugh.
"If I feel ill, I will double my labor.
"If I feel fear, I will plunge ahead.
"If I feel inferior, I will wear new garments.
"If I feel uncertain, I will raise my voice.
"If I feel poverty, I will think of wealth to come.
"If I feel incompetent, I will think of past success.
"If I feel insignificant, I will remember my goals.
"Today, I will be the master of my emotions."

– Og Mandino

Let me say again, with emphasis – I am not a doctor, psychologist, scientist, licensed counselor, psychiatrist, medical researcher, nurse, physician's assistant, or anything of the sort.

For that reason, I cannot be so bold as to prescribe a hard-and-fast solution to your depression. I cannot and will not say whether medication is or is not the answer. For some, it very well may be. For some, it reportedly works great. I've been told that finding the right drug works miracles. Bravo and hallelujah. That's what I was always looking for – a miracle cure.

Give me a happy pill.

For people like me, however, medication does not seem to produce noticeable results. Simply put, it just does not do anything, **in my experience.**

About six months ago, I guess, I stopped taking the fifth different anti-depressant prescribed to me over the past 10 or so years by a general practitioner. You know, the good ol' family doctor who looks in your ears, down your throat, and runs a stethoscope over your chest and back while asking you to take another deep breath before you've had a chance to completely inhale and exhale the first one.

That's what those guys and gals do – they try one of an assortment of the most popular pills, and if that works, great. If it doesn't, try another. If that one doesn't work, maybe try a different one.

I never really felt any different taking any of the medications prescribed to me, so why take them?

I am not an expert, but I can say – strictly my own opinion – that we are an over-medicated society. Pharmaceuticals is a tremendous money machine and doctors are part of the system. Many are quick to whip out the ol' prescription pad for just about everything. It is what they are trained to do.

According to some sources, in 2015, the United States was the largest single pharmaceutical market in the world, producing more than $400 billion in revenue. Europe generated around $200 billion in American dollars.

If you ask me, and I apologize to all the good-intentioned medical professionals everywhere, the purpose of medical care today is mostly to treat symptoms, instead of actual disease prevention and cure.

But I digress once again ….

Hell, if I could take a pill every day and feel better, walk around on cloud nine all the time, smiling and happy, I'd probably do it. I'm sure I would. But that has never happened.

I can't tell you what to do. I can only share my experiences, my knowledge, my research, and encourage you to find out what works best for you.

One thing I do strongly believe is the old adage that says happiness is an inside job.

If you are looking to people, places and things to make you happy, I can tell you for a fact that you are looking the wrong way. Barking up the wrong tree, as it were.

You know that person looking back at you in the mirror this morning when you brushed your teeth? That's the only person in this world who can make you truly happy.

For me, one of the big keys to happiness is learning to live one day at a time. Sure, it's a cliché, but it is so true.

So true, but not something I have ever come close to mastering. Living life one day at a time, savoring the moment, enjoying every day as it comes, being grateful for the little things, forgetting about the past and not worrying about the future, is something that has never come naturally to me.

Not even close.

In my mind, this is something that requires consistent, regular practice, which is something I have never had the discipline to do, even though I know I should do it, and want to do it.

Instead, I'm an all-pro at living in the past and projecting into the future – sometimes all at the same time – while neglecting to just relax and enjoy today.

Today is all we have, folks.

Yesterday is gone. Whatever happened cannot be changed, no matter how hard you try. Tomorrow is some sort of illusion that has not even happened yet. Planning for the future is one thing, but worrying about it is crazy, y'all.

Listen, we only get one life, for heaven's sakes, and I've spent way too much of mine perfecting the art of being miserable. Don't you do it, too.

There was never a conscious decision on my part to be unhappy – I don't enjoy feeling bad – but just a lot of going about things all wrong. Let me count the ways:

o   Comparing myself to others.
o   Worrying too much about what other people think.
o   Mind-reading (*imagining* what other people think).
o   People-pleasing; wanting *everyone* to like me.
o   Re-living the past again and again and again.
o   Worrying about the future.
o   Not accepting reality; wishing or even pretending things were different than they really are.
o   Taking criticism to heart (the old sticks and stones thing).
o   Beating myself up over mistakes, bad decisions.

Whew, quite a list.

Now, let's add fear to the equation.

Fear is a big one. Fear has always been a driving factor in my insanity, my crazy monkey brain stinkin' thinkin'. I don't like to admit that I'm scared of anything, but I most certainly am. Not so much fearful of physical things, although there are some of those, but mostly emotional fears – fear of rejection; fear of humiliation; fear of being alone.

Now, don't get me wrong. I enjoy my solitude. I don't mind being alone, spending time by myself. In fact, a lot of times, I prefer it. But not on a permanent basis, twenty-four hours a day, seven days a week.

As a man obviously filled with contradictions, I shy away from social activities whenever I can, but I also inevitably have a good time when I do suck it up and show my face somewhere. My wife always tells me she marvels at how easily I am able to talk to people, and how she watches me sometimes and how I seem to make whomever I am talking to feel important, that I'm really interested in them and what they have to say.

And I am, for the most part, interested in them and what they have to say. People and their lives are fascinating to me.

One thing I've always been fearful of is turning out like my father. He's a good man, but he is pretty much self-absorbed, mostly friendless, negative about everything, and definitely not a happy camper. Not to mention broken down physically. Years of neglect and all that negativity caused a lot of those health problems, I imagine.

I think I also have a pretty profound fear of death, although I don't like to admit that, either. I went to a fire and brimstone church from around age seven to fifteen, and I grew up thinking God was going to get me, punish me. The way I see it, there is nothing at all loving about a creator who sends you down to such a beautiful and screwed-up planet, keeps track of all your transgressions, and then sends you to burn in hell after you die and report back to heaven for a debriefing on how things went.

One way I have tried to overcome my fear of death is through researching and writing a book, "Destination Unknown: What Happens to Us When We Die?" I spent several months interviewing people from all over the world – face to face, by phone, Skype, e-mail – and asking them two basic questions: are they afraid of dying, and what do they think happens when they die. The answers were fascinating, and the book turned out pretty well.

I didn't really learn anything I didn't already know, but it was interesting to hear a variety of different viewpoints.

One thing I strongly suggest you do is join my private Facebook support group. Being part of a circle of like-minded people offering encouragement, sympathy and support is never a bad thing. Nobody understands depression and anxiety like a fellow sufferer.

I have fairly recently met two amazing people – one male; one female – who suffer from depression, and there was an instant connection, a bond, the first time I sat with them and talked. I can literally tell them anything, and they get it. They know. They don't judge; don't think I'm crazy; don't cringe at the mention of ugly stuff. They understand things most people do not.

At the end of this book, I have included some bonus material on such topics as: how to recognize depression, signs and symptoms; what to do about depression and anxiety; natural approaches to treating depression without using medication; dietary approaches to depression; and more.

I truly hope, with all my heart and soul, that you find something in these pages that helps you.

In the end, it is up to you, really, to find a way to get happy. Just like I wrote in the introduction to this book, the chances of somebody coming along, wrapping you in their loving arms, and magically changing you from sad to happy, are not good. Making a change is up to you.

You can do it.

Yes, you can.

Please, don't give up.

"Don't Quit"

by John Greenleaf Whittier

When things go wrong as they sometimes will,
When the road you're trudging seems all up hill,
When the funds are low and the debts are high,
And you want to smile, but you have to sigh.
When care is pressing you down a bit,
Rest if you must, but don't you quit.
Life is strange, with its twists and turns
As every one of us sometimes learns;
And many a failure comes about
When he might have won, had he stuck it out;
Don't give up though the pace seems slow –
You may succeed with another blow.
Success is failure turned inside out –
The silver tint of the clouds of doubt,
And you never can tell just how close you are,
It may be near when it seems so far;
So stick to the fight when you're hardest hit –
It's when things seem worst that you must not quit.

Things to look for

Depression can be a tricky thing. Here are some characteristics that might indicate you or someone else might be one of the "lucky" ones:

Persistent negative thinking:
> Feeling hopeless.
> Thoughts of 'why bother.'
> Feeling like things are always going wrong.
> Failure to see the positive side of difficult situations.
> Excessive guilt or shame.
> Extreme self-criticism.

Decreased activity or energy level:
> Constant fatigue.
> Decrease or cessation of previously enjoyed exercise.
> Restlessness; agitation.
> Lack of stamina; getting tired easily.

Changes in mood:
> Unusually short temper.
> Mood swings.
> Crying for no reason.
> Feeling agitated; unable to relax.
> Constant frustration.
> Unusual aggression.

Lost interest:
> Giving up favorite hobbies and activities.
> Feeling detached from the world.
> Avoiding others, including loves ones.
> Declining social engagements.
> Neglecting everyday responsibilities.
> Declining sexual activity.

Foggy brain:
> Hard to concentrate.
> Difficulty remembering things.
> Unusual forgetfulness.

Problems focusing on routine tasks.

Trouble sleeping:

Hard to fall asleep.

Frequent waking up through the night.

Sleeping longer than usual.

Appetite changes:

Loss of interest in food.

Missing meals.

Emotional eating.

Eating disorders.

Physical changes:

Ongoing aches and pains.

Excessive, unusual stress.

Increase in self-medicating.

Self-destructive behavior:

Excessive alcohol consumption.

Abusing drugs.

Risky sexual activity.

Taking unusual risks.

Thoughts about death:

Preoccupation with dying.

Thinking about ways to kill yourself.

Sudden concern with getting personal affairs in order.

If any of this sounds familiar, it may be time to seek help.

Recognizing and admitting to a problem is the most difficult and important part of recovery. Like I said before, admitting you have a problem and asking for help is not a sign of weakness, but just the opposite. It is a sign of strength and courage.

So go ahead. If you see yourself or someone you care about in any of those categories, take the next step and get some help. Make an appointment with a doctor for a checkup, then tell him or her exactly what is going on, and take it from there.

Things can and will get better.

A Natural Approach

Medication may be the answer for some people, but depression may also be the product of a negative, destructive environment. A learned behavior. A negative mindset, and generally lousy outlook on life. The mind is a powerful thing.

I think that is mostly the case with me. I learned negative thinking from birth – possibly in the womb – and have practiced it most of my life. I never learned what it means to love myself, to be proud of myself and my accomplishments, to realize that it's okay to make mistakes, and that I don't have to be perfect to be a good person.

Changing old habits is not easy. I have changed some of my lifelong negative thinking patterns, but I still have a ways to go. Here are some suggestions from experts that I plan to incorporate into my daily life, as I keep working to improve myself:

• Learning "mindfulness": this involves living in the moment, not thinking about the past or the future. Dwelling on stupid shit from last week, last month, last year – or in my case, as far back as high school – doesn't do a damn bit of good. Is it going to change anything? Is worrying about what might happen in the future going to do any good today, right now? No! The future is a fantasy, and the vast majority of things we worry about never actually happen, anyway.

I have a handmade poster on my wall at work that I don't look at often enough. Here's what it says:

"If you are feeling overwhelmed by life, come back to the present moment, the here and now, forget about everything else, look around you and simply savor all that is beautiful and comforting. Now, take a deep breath and just relax."

• Using touch: Studies indicate that "touch therapy" may help in managing or overcoming depression, lowering the stress-produced hormone cortisol, and increasing oxytocin, a "feel-good" hormone that some say makes us not only feel better, but also live longer and happier lives. So what is touch therapy? Simple. Things like massage, reiki, acupuncture, and reflexology.

I have experience with all those things, and that experience has always been positive.

A good, hour-long massage is heaven on Earth. Health experts say that up to ninety percent of disease is stress-related, and one of the purposes of massage therapy is to manage and relieve stress. I'm here to tell you, it works great.

Instead of being considered as some sort of luxury item, massage is actually a therapeutic, and some say necessary, way to maintain good health. If money is an issue, look around and you can find something affordable. Find a massage school; they offer great rates and I have friends who rave about them.

- <u>Cut out negative self-talk</u>: This is one of the big ones for me. I don't talk badly about myself as much as I used to, but I still have a lot of negative self-thought. I think negative things sometimes – I just don't verbalize them. Really, it's the same thing, though, isn't it?

Again, old habits die hard, but one way to deal with negative self-talk is to be aware of the fact that you do it. When it happens, don't take yourself seriously. Remember, your thinking patterns are coming from a depressed person, so do not give those negative ideas any credence. See them for what they are, and let it go. You don't have to believe them. You can even talk to those thoughts – no, I'm not an idiot; hey, I did my best and next time I'll do better; you're wrong, I am a good person.

- <u>Distract yourself</u>: When you start to get into that stinkin' thinkin', take your butt somewhere and do something different. Go for a walk, play fetch with the dog, mow the lawn, take a swim, ride a bicycle, straighten up that cluttered garage – do something active to get your mind out of its fear and worry mode.

One of the best times of my life was walking the Camino de Santiago, six to eight hours a day, seven days a week, for a month. While I was there, someone explained to me that the human body is designed for walking; it likes to walk. There is a route I've mapped out that starts at my driveway, winds through my little neighborhood, along a two-lane county road for a while, then back through another neighborhood and around to my driveway again, a total of right around four miles.

I have a pretty quick walking pace, and I finish it in about an hour. A great way to relive some tension, distract yourself, and get in a decent little workout. Highly recommended by yours truly.

• <u>Call or visit a friend</u>: When I get wrapped up in the funk, I tend to isolate myself. Stay locked up in the house. But when I do get up and get out, it always works wonders, and you never know what might happen. I went to a little backyard party a while back – didn't want to go; wife basically forced me – where I met a new friend who also suffers from depression (a lot worse case than mine), and that led to meeting a female friend of his who also suffers from severe depression.

I have not known either one of these people for very long, but there was an instant connection the first time we sat together and talked. They understand perfectly what I go through sometimes. If I had stayed holed up in the house instead of going to that party, I'd have never met either one of them. Sometimes, things happen for a reason.

Pick one of your most positive friends and give them a call. Invite them over for coffee, out to lunch, or something.

• <u>Journaling</u>: not hard to imagine I'd be a proponent of writing down your thoughts. I do it all the time. Sometimes, I use it in my writing, and sometimes I write in a notebook just to get things out in the open. Problems look a whole lot smaller on paper than they seem when they're swimming around inside your head.

Something I started two weeks ago, as I worked on wrapping up this book, is keeping a gratitude journal. I put the day's date at the top of a clean sheet of paper in a regular spiral notebook, and I write this: "Why is today a good day?" Then, I answer the question.

Here's an actual excerpt from a page in my gratitude journal:

"Why is today a good day?

"Well, first of all, it was a better than average weekend. Every weekend is a good one, but some are better than others.

"I worked with a guy a long time ago named Marvin, who was probably in his late thirties, was bald on top, wore thick eyeglasses, had a big, blonde moustache, unbuttoned his shirts halfway down to show off the assortment of gold chains he wore around his neck, and carried a thick wad of one-dollar bills wrapped in a twenty to try and impress the ladies.

"Marvin was on the bad end of a messy divorce and had some issues. One thing he was fond of saying was: 'Weekends are like sex – the worst I ever had was fantastic.' Okay, so he was kind of a pig, but I always thought that was funny.

"One thing great about this past weekend was reconnecting with my youngest daughter, Katy. We haven't seen much of each other the past few months, although we live about fifteen miles apart. We had breakfast Sunday, and had a great time. I saw her new apartment and gave her my grandfather's old desk to put in her bedroom.

"She is doing really well, and we promised to not let so much time pass between visits anymore."

Get yourself some sort of notebook and start a journal. Write down things that are bothering you, or things that are making you feel good. Write down a couple of things every day for which you are thankful, grateful. Write about things that happen in your day that made you smile or lifted your mood.

Try it – you'll like it.

• Never give up: Look, one of the signs of depression is thinking about suicide. My grandfather committed suicide, and I know other people who have done it. But here's the deal – no matter what, I kinda want to hang around and see how the story ends. You know what I mean? I don't really want giving up to be the end of my life story. Hang in there. You never know what tomorrow may bring.

Exercise for Depression

This is something I badly need to work on – getting more exercise.

I used to work out every morning, five days a week, in the gym: lifting weights, walking and running on the treadmill, the exercise bike. I was in great shape, lean and muscular, looked good and felt good.

Now, I neither look good nor feel good. I'm probably thirty-five pounds heavier than I was back in those days, and I don't even want to think about what my body-fat percentage might be now. I know I've traded a lot of lean muscle mass for flabby, fat mass.

I don't like the way I look, and that has to affect the way I feel about myself, and the way I feel mentally in general. I'm basically an active person – I enjoy moving, being outdoors, using my body, sweating, feeling that good ol' muscle soreness that comes with a strenuous workout – but I've turned into a slug. I don't think slugs are very happy.

And get this – some studies have shown that exercise can be as effective in treating depression as medication.

A good, hard workout can trigger your body to release something called endorphins, which react in your brain to offset your perception of pain. These endorphins also can trigger a positive feeling throughout the body, similar to the powerful drug morphine. That is why people sometimes describe feeling "euphoric," happy, excited, after a strenuous workout – sometimes referred to as a runner's high.

One time, many years ago, following a good, hard run of about three miles, I stopped at the mailboxes in my apartment complex to check my mail, and as I stood there, I got this massive rush from head to toe that felt really, really good. Nothing that intense ever happened again, and I'm not sure why it did that time, but I know for a fact that runner's high is a real thing.

So, what to do?

Sure, if you're depressed, feeling bad about yourself and the world, it can be tough to just get up off the couch, not to mention actually doing something like exercise. If you need to, take it slow. One step at a time. Go for a walk around the block. That's it. If that's all you can manage, that's fine. Just do it. Do something. The next day, go do it again. See if you can make it twice around the block.

Maybe the most important thing about exercise – and I know this one from experience – is consistency. You have to figure out a schedule, and stick to it.

Number one, if you are hit-and-miss about it, the results will be slow in coming, and you're likely to get discouraged and quit. Number two, every time you skip a day, it makes it that much easier to say screw it, and skip the next day, too. Pretty soon, you're skipping every day again.

One really good suggestion is to find a workout partner. You can help motivate each other. There were times I wanted to stay home and sleep in for another hour, but I knew my partner would be there waiting for me, and I didn't want to let him down.

If you have the means, join a gym, enroll in an exercise class, hire a personal trainer. All good ways to motivate yourself, and hold yourself accountable.

For something like walking, you can do that every day. Maybe take Sundays off, but no more than one day. When you're talking about something more strenuous, like lifting weights, I used to work out Monday, Tuesday, Thursday and Friday at the gym, and do something like an hour on the treadmill on Wednesdays, along with abdominal exercises, like crunches, leg lifts, sit-ups.

Most importantly, find an activity that you enjoy. I am not a big fan of running these days. I'm a good runner, and it's great exercise, but it's just not any fun. I tend to believe in the old adage that says: "I never saw someone jogging with a big smile on their face." It's just really not my thing.

I love walking, and long walks can be a great workout. Throw on a backpack with fifteen-twenty pounds of stuff inside it, and the workout gets even better.

Here is a list of activities you might consider:

- Walking. A ten-minute walk can reportedly improve your mood for two hours.
- Hiking (if you have some nature trails, or a lake or a river nearby, even better).
- Jogging.
- Yoga.
- Tai-chi.
- Gardening – hey, don't knock it if you haven't tried it. There's something very therapeutic about getting down, digging in the dirt, connecting with the Earth and the soil, feeling it, working it, planting beautiful things and seeing them grow.
- Bicycle riding.
- Crank up some music and dance around the house.
- Take the dog for a walk.
- Use stairs instead of an elevator.
- Park your car at the far end of the parking lot. In Texas, we like to find a shady spot to park our pickups, especially in the heat of summer. Problem is, if that shady spot is under a tree, birds will quickly organize a target practice.

Whatever you decide, just do something. To be safe, check with your doctor before starting a new exercise program. If you're a little older, like me, you may think you can still get out there and run around like you're 25 years old, but your body will most likely tell you different.

So go check with the doc, then get your butt off the couch and go outside.

You got this …

Diet for Depression

Some research suggests that diet and depression may be related. Studies have indicated that people with poor eating habits – a diet filled with such things as processed meats, sugar, and fried foods – are more likely to report symptoms of depression.

On the other hand, people with a diet containing lots of fish, fruits and vegetables may be less likely to report being depressed. Additionally, this type of diet also leads to fewer cases of such things as Alzheimer's disease, diabetes, and heart disease.

Junk food is called junk food for a reason.

I have eaten so much junk in my life, it's ridiculous. A guy who works at our local golf course started losing weight like crazy, and of course, everybody was commenting about it, so when I asked him one time how he was doing it, he wouldn't say much: "You know, diet and exercise."

A few months later, I must have caught him on a more talkative day, because this time when I asked, he said this: "Here's what I do. If it comes out of a window, I don't eat it."

In other words, no drive-throughs. No fast food. This guy had to have lost at least fifty pounds, mostly by cutting out junk food.

One thing you really need to watch, as far as helping with depression, is eating too many sweets and highly-refined carbohydrates, like breads and pastas made from white flour, for example. These things wreak havoc with your blood sugar levels, making them spike and then plummet, leading to sometimes tremendous mood swings.

Artificial sweeteners and soft drinks are terrible for your body. Stay away from that stuff. There are plenty of alternatives.

Processed foods. All those chemical additives and preservatives aren't good for anything except making the giant food companies rich. Along with my friend Mike's suggestion about not eating anything that is handed to you through a window, here's another one from me: "If it comes in a box, don't eat it."

There are other things that experts warn against, like caffeine, alcohol, canned foods with high sodium content, but if you can get away from the fast food, sugar, refined carbs, sodas and processed foods, you'll go a long way toward improving not only your mental health, but your physical health, as well.

Something also reported to help with depression is folate (folic acid), a B vitamin naturally occurring in beans such as pinto, garbanzo and black beans.

Other dietary sources of folate include such things as eggs, broccoli, avocado, asparagus, spinach, and tomato juice.

A study published in the Journal of Clinical Psychiatry reported that depressed patients showed improvement in mood when they were given omega-3 supplements. As with folic acid, these omega-3 fatty acids help strengthen brain neurotransmitters including serotonin, a mood regulator. Our bodies don't produce omega-3s on their own, so supplementation or food is the only way to get them. The most common source is fish: salmon, sardines, mackerel, herring, albacore tuna, as well as flaxseed and walnuts.

Do a little research.

Find out what can work for you.

Practice Optimism

You are the master of your emotions.

Good, bad, or indifferent. You have the power to manage what goes on inside your head.

None of us is a mindless protoplasm, simply oozing around reacting to outside stimuli. Things happen throughout the day that affect us, of course. Something happens at work that causes anger or frustration. Somebody cuts us off in traffic. Something disappointing happens, and we feel sadness. We receive an unexpected bit of good news, and now we feel happy.

That is not how it should be.

We humans have the intellectual capacity to respond in ways that can make things worse or make things better.

Shit happens, y'all. Some shit is bad, and some shit is good. What matters is how you deal with the shit that comes your way.

What is that old saying … ten percent of life is what happens, and ninety percent is how I react to the things that happen? Something like that.

Psychologists say we can regulate our emotions, or "dysregulate" them. Get some bad news and feel sad? Of course. Sitting around and crying about it for a week is a different story. The trick is to acknowledge that, sure, we feel sad and that is perfectly normal, but then to take steps to feel better.

Sounds to me like some positive self-talk, instead of the negative kind. And we've already talked about that, haven't we?

I wrote a book a while back titled, "30-Day Optimism Solution: How to Change from Pessimist to Optimist in 30 Days or Less." It is the story of my own month-long challenge to change my lifelong habit of negative thinking. You can find it here: www.johnhenryiii.com/my-books.

Although I've gotten a lot better at being more positive, I have a long way to go. Breaking a lifelong habit is not such an easy thing.

Quantum physics tells us that our thoughts have an actual frequency and unique vibration that attracts similar frequencies. In other words, negative thinking attracts negative energy, while positive thinking attracts positive energy. It is said that our thoughts have a profound effect on our subconscious mind, a powerful part of the human psyche which basically works very hard to make our thoughts come true.

For that reason, our mood is greatly affected by our subconscious mind.

Listen, I'm no expert, but I've done some studying on the power of the subconscious. Mainly in the area of golf. Yes, golf.

But I don't play golf, you say. Doesn't matter. This is still an excellent way to demonstrate the power of the subconscious mind.

Have you ever heard that we humans only use ten percent of our brain power? Well, that is sort of true. We only use ten percent of our conscious brain power. The other ninety percent involves subconscious brain activity.

Do you have to tell your heart to beat? Are you conscious of your breathing on a minute-to-minute basis? Do you have to remind your eyes to blink, or your body to release certain hormones at the right time? All those things are happening subconsciously, right?

Here is the way the subconscious mind supposedly works in golf:

You are faced with a shot over a water hazard, for example, or over a sand trap, or into a narrow tree-lined fairway. If you tell yourself, "Don't hit it in the water," or "Don't hit it in the sand," or "Don't hit it in the woods," your subconscious mind does not hear the word "don't." All it hears is "hit it in the water," or "hit it in the sand," or "hit it in the trees." And it does its dead-level best to help you accomplish the mission.

Here's another example:

If I tell you, "Don't think about a steaming, freshly baked pizza coming out of the oven. Don't imagine the steam rising off the bubbling cheese and the moist pepperoni."

You just thought about that pizza, didn't you? Maybe even got a little hungry. You can't *not* think about it. That's how our mind works.

That is why you have to be careful about the information you feed into your subconscious. If you put negative stuff in there, your subconscious mind absorbs it, stores it away, and believes it. A subconscious mind filled with negativity tends to produce an overall negative outlook on life. When you speak negatively about yourself, your subconscious accepts it, and pretty soon it becomes part of your psyche.

This is why it is so important to eliminate the negative self-talk.

Fill your mind with positive thoughts.

I read somewhere a story about a tightrope walker, like one of those people in the circus. Someone asked this guy how he was able to accomplish something that seemed so difficult and dangerous. He said the secret is simple: "Don't look down."

Keep your eyes up, and focused on where you want to go. Where the eyes go, the body will follow.

This is true for a lot of things in life.

I took a motorcycle safety course one time, when I thought I was going to become one of those middle-aged weekend bikers, looking all cool in the leather jacket, boots, sunglasses and do-rag. One of the things they teach you about maneuvering a motorcycle is to always look where you want to go, and your body – and the bike – will take you there. Don't look at where you are, but at where you want to go. Around a curve, for example. Don't look at the curve, look past the curve to the road ahead. That is where you want to go.

My 10-month motorcycle riding career ended after a minor crash and two parking lot drops, when I failed to heed that simple instruction. Heading around a double-ess curve at 60 mph, I swung out a little too wide in the second portion of the curve, saw myself heading toward a large ditch alongside the elevated roadway, and instead of looking ahead, keeping my focus on the pavement ahead of the curve, I focused on the ditch. And that's exactly where I wound up. Luckily, I didn't get seriously injured, but the bike was a total loss – it went end over end, sailing over my head as I slid for what seemed like forever on my ass, and then rolled several times before coming to a stop.

Along with helping ease depression, positive thinking may have other health-related benefits, as well. One study showed that adults with a family history of heart disease were half as likely to suffer a heart attack or other serious problems if they also had a positive attitude. The research suggested that people who exercise the power of positive thinking produce lower levels of stress hormones, which tends to help protect them against disease.

I have a close friend who has mastered the art of optimism. He has practiced positivity his whole life, over and over and over, on a daily basis, until it comes second nature to him. I asked Bobby if he ever has a bad day. He said, "No. Never." And he meant it. I said, "How the hell do you do that?" Here's what he said:

"Every morning, as soon as I wake up, the first thing I do – the very first thing – is I say, 'Today is going to be a great day.'"

I thought he was bullshitting me, but he was completely serious. He told me to try it. So I did.

Guess what?

It really does work. I don't do it every day – lately, I've been trying to form the habit of saying it every morning, as soon as I shut off that damn alarm clock – but on the days I say out loud, "Today is going to be a great day," I'm here to tell you that the day goes a whole lot better. It really does.

When I wrote my book on optimism, I asked Bobby to write the foreword. Here it is:

"My dear friend, John, asked me to write the forward to his new book. An honor. He asked me to discuss, describe and define the keys to happiness born of the power of positive thinking. As I began to dwell upon this request, a simple thought occurred to me – what sets us apart from all other living creatures is the ability to think and use thought to form decisions, ideas, strategies and actions.

"However, this same 'power' can also work against us in the form of small thinking, negativity, depression or distress. What we see is what we get. How we think is what determines our reality.

"I know, I know, we've heard it all before in various ways. Words can be powerful but words alone cannot change a thing. We have to learn how to view life differently. See things in different 'words.' Every day is a brand new day. A new beginning. It is a blank piece of paper on which we get the chance to write a new story.

"My problem was that I would always write a story where I was the hero. I have found, over time, that I gain my true strength and happiness by uplifting others. I challenge you to discover and uncover that element of life that you've never seen before that already exists deep down inside of you. There are 86,400 seconds in a day. Any one of those could change the direction of your life.

"Think big thoughts. Grand thoughts. Always dream big. Throw your thoughts and dreams out there, but don't just sit and stare at them. Follow them and pick them up where they land and then, throw them out again. If you stay focused and keep repeating the process, you may not achieve your dream in *your* timing, but when you look back, you will see all the ground you have covered. That is the definition of achievement and success.

"The power of positive thinking."

Those are words from a master, and someone who has parlayed his efforts at positive thinking (and helping others) into a not-so-small fortune. He still sends me positive messages, YouTube videos, and other things on a regular basis, trying to inspire me and help me keep on keepin' on.

There are lots of ways and recommendations for how to practice and cultivate a habit of positive thinking. Here is a fairly short and simple system you can try:

Work on an attitude of gratitude. That's it.

An attitude of gratitude.

Being truly grateful is said to increase not only positive emotions and outlook on life, but may even improve physical health, as well.

One thing I did during my experiment to practice optimism was writing quotations on index cards, and posting them around the house. A few on the refrigerator; a few more on the bathroom mirror; a few on the visor of my pickup where I can see them.

Here are a few quotes to get you started:

"Live more; think less." – Sig Christenson.

"Once you replace negative thoughts with positive ones, you'll start having positive results." – Willie Nelson.

"We can complain because rose bushes have thorns, or rejoice because thorn bushes have roses." – Abraham Lincoln.

"Keep your face to the sunshine and you cannot see a shadow." – Helen Keller

"You are essentially who you create yourself to be, and all that occurs in your life is the result of your own making." – Stephen Richards

"Live life to the fullest, and focus on the positive." – Matt Cameron

"Your attitude is like a box of crayons that color your world. Constantly color your picture gray, and your picture will always be bleak. Try adding some bright colors to the picture by including humor, and your picture begins to lighten up." – Allen Klein

"If you're not making mistakes, then you're not doing anything. I'm positive that a doer makes mistakes." – John Wooden

"Positive thinking will let you do everything better than negative thinking will." – Zig Ziglar

"You cannot have a positive life and a negative mind." – Joyce Meyer.

"When you wake up every day, you have two choices. You can either be positive or negative; an optimist or a pessimist. I choose to be an optimist. It's all a matter of perspective." – Harvey Mackay.

"Believe that life is worth living and your belief will help create the fact." – William James.

Be good to yourself.

You are worth it; you deserve it.

You are not alone

You may recall me telling you to remember that in this struggle with depression, you are never alone?

Well, here is just a small sampling, in no particular order, of notable people throughout history who reportedly suffer or have suffered a similar condition as you and I.

Some made it; some didn't.

Most did quite well.

The actual list is much longer:

John Adams - Hans Christian Anderson - Abraham Lincoln
Brian Wilson - Winston Churchill - Mike Wallace
Ernest Hemingway - Buzz Aldrin - J.K. Rowling
Johnny Carson - William Blake - Terry Bradshaw
Truman Capote - Ray Charles - Woody Allen
Eric Clapton - Marilyn Monroe - Charles Dickens
William Faulkner - Harrison Ford - Stephen King
John Lennon - David Letterman - Michelangelo
Wolfgang Amadeus Mozart -   Isaac Newton
Charles M. Schulz - Mark Twain - Robin Williams
Oprah Winfrey - Isaac Asimov - Billy Joel
Walt Whitman - Calvin Coolidge - Art Buchwald
Charles Darwin - Emily Dickinson - Bob Dylan
Paul Getty - Audrey Hepburn - Vladimir Horowitz
Anthony Hopkins - Dwayne Johnson - Jack Kerouac
Meriwether Lewis - John Denver - Dolly Parton
John D. Rockefeller - Tennessee Williams

Quotes about depression

"Depression is like a wave. We all need to learn how to ride it and stay positive. Life can be hard but we can make it through with a smile." – source unknown

"Mental pain is less dramatic than physical pain, but it is more common and also more hard to bear. The frequent attempt to conceal mental pain increases the burden: it is easier to say, 'My tooth is aching,' than to say, 'My heart is broken.'" – C.S. Lewis

"The mind is everything. What you think, you become." – Buddha

"Depression is the most unpleasant thing I have ever experienced … it is that absence of being able to envisage that you will ever be cheerful again. The absence of hope. That very deadened feeling, which is so very different from feeling sad. Sad hurts, but it's a healthy feeling. It is a necessary thing to feel. Depression is very different." – J.K. Rowling

"I'll never forget how the depression and loneliness felt good and bad at the same time. Still does." – Henry Rollins

"You largely constructed your depression. It wasn't given to you. Therefore, you can deconstruct it." – Albert Ellis

"It is never too late to be what you might have been." – George Eliot

"You say you're depressed – all I see is resilience. You are allowed to feel messed up and inside out. It doesn't mean you're defective – it just means you're human." – David Mitchell

"Bless your uneasiness as a sign that there is still life in you." – Dag Hammarskjold

"Every man has his secret sorrows which the world knows not; and often times we call a man cold when he is only sad." — Henry Wadsworth Longfellow

"When you're lost in those woods, it sometimes takes you a while to realize that you are lost. For the longest time, you can convince yourself that you've just wandered off the path, that you'll find your way back to the trailhead any moment now. Then night falls again and again, and you still have no idea where you are, and it's time to admit that you have bewildered your-self so far off the path that you don't even know which direction the sun rises anymore." – Elizabeth Gilbert

"You know all that sympathy that you feel for an abused child who suffered without a good mom or dad to love and care for them? Well, they don't stay children forever. No one magically becomes an adult the day they turn eighteen. Some people grow up sooner; many grow up later. Some never really do. But just remember that some people in this world are older versions of those same kids we cry for." – Ashly Lorenzana

"No matter what form of depression you may suffer from, love and acceptance are the two essential elements necessary in developing control over your symptoms ..." — Amy Weintraub

"Our greatest glory is not in never falling, but in rising every time we fall." – Confucius

"Depression is the common cold of the deluded human being. And according to Buddha, all human beings are quite deluded." – Stephen Cope

"When you're surrounded by all these people, it can be lonelier than when you are by yourself. You can be in a huge crowd, but if you don't feel like you can trust anyone or talk to anybody, you feel like you're really alone." – Fiona Apple

"If you know someone who's depressed, please resolve never to ask them why. Depression isn't a straightforward response to a bad situation; depression just is – like the weather. Try to understand the blackness ... be there for them when they come through the other side. It's hard to be a friend to someone who is depressed, but it is one of the kindest, noblest and best things you will ever do." – Stephen Fry

"There are two ways to live your life. One is as though nothing is a miracle. The other is as though everything is a miracle." – Albert Einstein

A Small Favor to Ask

Thanks for reading this important book. I hope you found something meaningful or helpful in some way. Now, please help me reach others who might benefit from hearing my story by taking just a minute to write a review of this book on Amazon. Your reviews mean a great deal to me, but more importantly, they really do help others find this book. You never know, your review might lead someone to discover an answer that changes their life for the better.

Take a minute now and go write that review.

About the author

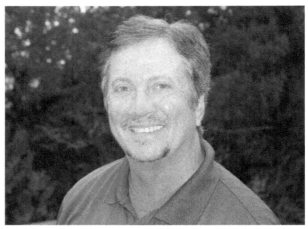

John Henry Clark III is an award-winning journalist, freelance writer, author, photographer, musician, artist, and avid golfer who was born and raised in Houston, Texas. He graduated with a degree in journalism from the University of Houston, and spent more than twenty years as a newspaper reporter and magazine writer for various publications throughout the Lone Star state.

The tragic death of his mother in June 2000 turned Clark's world upside down, and he began to re-assess his priorities and consider a career change. After much soul-searching and consideration, he decided to take his lifelong love for learning and become a public school English teacher. Along with providing an exciting new challenge, teaching school also gave him time during the summer months to pursue a long-awaited project to research and write a book describing what people believe about God and why they believe whatever they believe.

That effort turned into his first published book, *Finding God: An Exploration of Diversity in America's Heartland*. A tireless seeker, researcher and questioner, John has written a number of other fascinating books dealing with the human experience, from tragedies to triumphs and more, including his best-selling *Camino: Laughter and Tears along Spain's 500-mile Camino de Santiago*.

FREE offer

Hey, guys and gals, listen up – since you've gotten this far, I want to make you an offer:

How about a free book? Yes, one of my books absolutely free.

It's one of my favorites: *Camino: Laughter and Tears Along Spain's 500-mile Camino de Santiago*, the story of my pilgrimage(s) across northern Spain. I've never been much of a traveler, and when I decided to go overseas for the first time … well, you'll have to read the story to find out.

Go right now and send an email to: depressionblues.net@gmail.com, let me know where to send your copy, and voila! it's yours.

C'mon, grab this special offer while it lasts.

You'll be glad you did.

Other works

To read more of Clark's books about depression and related issues, along with information on how to receive his monthly newsletter, podcast, videos, and other special offers, go to www.depressionblues.net.

A complete listing of all his book titles is also available at www.johnhenryiii.com.

Sign his mailing list at: www.johnclarkbooks.com

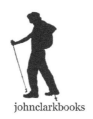

johnclarkbooks

www.depressionblues.net
www.johnclarkbooks.com
www.johnhenryiii.com

CPSIA information can be obtained
at www.ICGtesting.com
Printed in the USA
LVHW03s1930050918
589229LV00017B/1531/P